"My Nerves Are Bad"

"My Nerves Are Bad"

Puerto Rican Women Managing Mental Illness and HIV Risk

Sana Loue

Vanderbilt University Press ■ Nashville

Nashville, Tennessee 37235

First printing 2011

This book is printed on acid-free paper
made from 30% post-consumer recycled content.
Manufactured in the United States of America

Library of Congress Cataloging-in-Publication Data

Loue, Sana.
"My nerves are bad" : Puerto Rican women managing
mental illness and HIV risk / Sana Loue.
p. ; cm.
Puerto Rican women managing mental illness and HIV risk
Includes bibliographical references and index.
ISBN 978-0-8265-1753-1 (cloth ed. : alk. paper)
ISBN 978-0-8265-1754-8 (pbk. ed. : alk. paper)
1. AIDS (Disease)—Ohio. 2. Mentally ill—Health and hygiene—Ohio.
3. Puerto Rican women—Health and hygiene—Ohio. 4. Puerto Rican
women—mental health—Ohio. I. Title. II. Title: Puerto Rican women
managing mental illness and HIV risk.
[DNLM: 1. HIV Infections—ethnology—Puerto Rico. 2. HIV
Infections—ethnology—United States. 3. Mental Disorders—
ethnology—Puerto Rico. 4. Mental Disorders—ethnology—United
States. 5. Health Policy—Puerto Rico. 6. Health Policy—United States.
7. Hispanic Americans—Puerto Rico. 8. Hispanic Americans—United
States. 9. Socioeconomic Factors—Puerto Rico. 10. Socioeconomic
Factors—United States. 11. Women's Health—Puerto Rico.
12. Women's Health—United States. WA 300 AA1]
RA643.84.O3L68 2011
362.196'9792009771—dc22
2010036853

God tells you not to worry about tomorrow
because tomorrow is not promised. The birds
don't have any clothes but God provides.
We are his children and he will provide.
Sometimes we feel sad because we are human,
but you ask God and you will feel better.

—Maria, diagnosed with schizophrenia
(quoted in Loue and Sajatovic 2006, p. 1175)

*Todos nacimos para morir. Dios nos lleva
cuando nos necesite.* [We are all born to
die. God takes us when he needs us.]

—Narcisa, diagnosed with bipolar disorder

Contents

Tables

Acknowledgments

This book could not have been written, and the study on which it is based could not have been conducted, without the generous support and encouragement of a multitude of people. First and foremost, it is impossible to convey accurately the debt owed to the women who were the participants in the study and are the personalities portrayed in this volume. Their names, as well as the names of their family members, friends, and providers, have been changed to safeguard their identities and protect their privacy. Street names and specific locations have also been modified. The women welcomed us into their lives, sometimes with enthusiasm and other times with reservations and suspicion, but welcomed us nevertheless. At times, it appeared to require of them an almost herculean effort to get past the paranoia of their mental illness and their fear that we would reject or judge them. A number of the women moved frequently during the course of the study, some to great distances from Cleveland, but, even so, they remained in contact with the study team, resumed participation upon their return, and contributed significantly to what we have learned.

Various institutions are to be thanked for their support. The National Institute of Mental Health provided the funding both for this study, R01 MH63016, and for its precursor study, R29 MH58070, which provided the impetus to examine specifically the context of HIV risk among Latinas with severe mental illness. My program officers for each of these grants, Dr. David Stoff and Dr. Willo Pequegnat, respectively, each contributed their enthusiasm and insight to the respective studies. My academic institution, Case Western Reserve University, provided me with the additional resources that made these studies possible. Several individuals, in particular, are to be thanked for their support and vision: Dr. Alfred Rimm, Dr. Nathan Berger, Dr. Ralph Horwitz, Ann Duli, and Edward Bruss.

Numerous agencies and private individuals participated on our Community Advisory Board, generously sharing their insights with us in matters relating to recruitment for the study, retention of participants, translation of instruments, and the interpretation of data. I list the northeast Ohio advisory board members here, with trepidation that I may have inadvertently omitted a member, and with the knowledge that some of them have since changed their organizational affiliations: Marco Cardona of the Cleveland Department of Health, the late Rev. David Fallon of San Juan Bautista Church, Maribel Garcia of the Cuyahoga County Department of Children and Family Services, Antonia Montijo of the Cleveland Police Department, Katherine O'Brien of the AIDS Taskforce of Greater Cleveland, Nidia Perez of the Center for Families and Children, Rafael Rivera, Jennifer Smith of Recovery Resources, and Luis Vázquez of Casa Alma. Neither the study nor this volume would have been possible without the dedication, insights, and energy of study co-investigators, collaborators, and staff. Dr. Martha Sajatovic provided significant guidance and training to staff members and has collaborated on various papers arising from this study. Nancy Mendez was the best project coordinator imaginable, often "debriefing" the ethnographers to help them process their own responses to the scenes that they had witnessed during the shadowing. The study could not have been possible without ethnographers Jenice Contreras and Ingrid Vargas, who brought their knowledge of northeast Ohio's Latino communities to the study and connected with the study participants and their family members to earn their trust. Transcription and data analysis were ably performed by Gary Edmunds and Anamaria Tejada, and by Emily Heaphy, who contributed to the statistical analysis for Chapter 8 of this volume.

Last, but certainly not least, I owe thanks to my editor, Michael Ames at Vanderbilt University Press. Michael offered excellent suggestions in response to earlier drafts of this volume, waiting patiently for the final version as I sifted through thousands of hours of transcripts to discern and then communicate a meaningful whole. Thanks are also owed to an anonymous reviewer, who provided excellent suggestions and insights.

A number of articles focusing on specific aspects of this study have been published in peer-reviewed scientific and health journals:

Friedman, S., and Loue, S. (2008). Intimate partner violence among women with severe mental illness. *Psychiatric Times, 25(4).*

Hatters-Friedman, S., and Loue, S. (2007). Incidence and prevalence of intimate partner violence by and against women with severe mental illness: A review. *Journal of Women's Health, 16(4)*, 471–80.

Hatters-Friedman, S., Loue, S., Heaphy, E., and Mendez, N. (2009). Partner violence victimization and perpetration by Puerto Rican women with severe mental illnesses. *Community Mental Health Journal.* doi:10.1007/s10597-009-9270-z (e-pub ahead of print).

Heaphy, E., and Loue, S. (2010). Comparing two approaches to acquiring HIV-risk data from Puerto Rican women with severe mental illness. *Journal of Immigrant and Minority Health, 12(1)*, 74–82.

Heaphy, E., Loue, S., Sajatovic, M., and Tisch, D. (2009). Impact of psychiatric and social characteristics on HIV sexual risk behavior in Puerto Rican women with severe mental illness. *Social Psychiatry and Psychiatric Epidemiology*. doi:10.1007/s00127-009-0146-x (e-pub ahead of print).

Loue, S. (2007). HIV prevention research among severely mentally ill Latinas: An examination of ethical issues in the context of gender and culture. *Acta Bioetica, 13(1)*, 81–97.

Loue S. (2006). Preventing HIV, eliminating disparities among Hispanics in the United States. *Journal of Immigrant and Minority Health, 8(4)*, 313–18.

Loue, S., and Mendez, N. (2006). "I don't know who I am": Severely mentally ill Latina WSW navigating differentness. *Journal of Lesbian Studies, 10(1/2)*, 249–66.

Loue, S., Mendez, N., and Sajatovic, M. (2008). Preliminary evidence for the integration of music into HIV prevention for severely mentally ill Latinas. *Journal of Immigrant and Minority Health, 10(6)*, 489–95.

Loue, S., and Sajatovic, M. (2008). Auditory and visual hallucinations in a sample of severely mentally ill Puerto Rican women: An examination of the cultural context. *Mental Health, Culture, and Religion, 11(6)*, 597–608.

Loue, S., and Sajatovic, M. (2008). Research with severely mentally ill Latinas: Successful recruitment and retention strategies. *Journal of Immigrant and Minority Health, 10(2)*, 145–53.

Loue, S., and Sajatovic, M. (2006). Spirituality, coping, and HIV risk and prevention in a sample of severely mentally ill Puerto Rican women. *Journal of Urban Health, 83(6)*, 1168–82.

Every effort was made to avoid duplication in this text of materials that have been previously published elsewhere. Any knowing duplication in the text is so noted by reference to the originally published work.

“My Nerves Are Bad”

1

Beyond Numbers

Faces of HIV and Mental Illness in Northeastern Ohio's Latino Communities

Katia was moving yet again. Born in Puerto Rico, she had come to the U.S. mainland while still a girl. She moved frequently within the city of Cleveland, essentially "couch surfing" from the home of one friend or sexual partner to another, attempting to put a roof over her head on the many nights when she did not have one of her own. She was often unemployed for all but brief periods of time, a result both of the symptoms of her bipolar disorder, which included visual and auditory hallucinations and suicidal ideation, and of her substance use, which centered on marijuana and the almost nightly ingestion of large quantities of alcohol but had also included LSD and cocaine. She had been sexually abused as a child and was frequently in relationships with abusive partners. Katia learned to support herself by trading sex for rent, car repairs, and various other necessities of life; by dancing in strip joints; by "shopping" from among the goods that well-heeled residents of better-appointed neighborhoods discarded at the curb as trash; and by relying on her social security benefits.

This time, her former lover Abe was helping her move. Isa, an ethnographer with the study that is the focus of this volume, had met Abe while visiting Katia. She had also met—and tripped over on several occasions—the alligator that lived in the soon-to-be oasis that Abe was constructing for it, now that he had finished jackhammering out the basement floor of his rented apartment. Katia nonchalantly provided Isa with an update on the alligator's well-being:

> He [Abe] is making a habitat downstairs for [his alligator]. He's big and doesn't fit in the tank anymore. You know the more space you give the alligator, the more they grow. [*Laughing*] Yes. He is going to be big as hell because they need room to grow. . . . He [Abe] had a snake before but his brother took it. The alligator escaped the other day but he found him downstairs eating rats. Can you imagine, he doesn't fit in that cage anymore. He wants him to grow real big. He holds him and everything.

Katia is only one of the fifty-three women who participated in the study that is the focus of this book. This is not, however, a story of mental illness, of Puerto Rican ethnicity, or of being female. It is, rather, a portrayal of life at the intersection of these various domains and identities, as the women navigate through the difficulties and challenges presented by seemingly unrelenting poverty, ubiquitous violence, sexism, fluctuating symptoms of mental illness, often unfathomable and unforgiving bureaucracies, and well-meaning, detached, and enabling social service providers. To a great degree, these fifty-three women remain marginalized both from larger, mainstream society and from the smaller communities and groups in which we live. They are labeled as "different"—so different, in fact, as to be considered deviant.[1] These are women who struggle with minority status as Puerto Ricans; with female status in a community dominated by men, and by subtle and not-so-subtle demands for women's conformity to a subservient role in male-female relationships; and with severe mental illness (bipolar disorder, major depression, or schizophrenia) in a world that demands full functioning and competence in all phases of life, at every moment. Some of these women must additionally struggle to maintain intimate partner relations with other women in what continues to be a heterosexist society.

Despite my best efforts to present accurately the events and exchanges that occurred, there remains the danger that the situation of these women will be romanticized, in much the same way that poverty and the attendant struggle to improve one's life are so often romanticized.[2] It is equally possible that readers will fault the women portrayed here for their lot in life, reflecting the widespread tendency to "blame the victim,"[3] or, at the other extreme, absolve the women of all responsibility for their choices and the ensuing consequences, thereby further disempowering them and disavowing the potential for positive change.

The story of my involvement with this community of Puerto Rican women began in 1997, with the submission of a grant application to the

National Institutes of Health (NIH) to examine HIV risk and prevention behaviors in a sample of Mexican men and women in San Diego County, California, and a sample of Puerto Rican men and women in Cuyahoga County, Ohio.[4] Participants for this first study were recruited from a wide range of sites, including housing projects, social service organizations, churches, vocational training programs, bodegas (small grocery stores), nightclubs, community clubs, and detention facilities. Because this was not a clinic-based sample, it came as a surprise to find, first, that 25 percent of the Puerto Rican women and 1 percent of the Mexican women reported that they had been diagnosed with a severe mental illness during the previous year and, second, that this subgroup of women participating in the study had the highest HIV risk behaviors among the female participants. Our data from that study do not tell us why a higher proportion of the Puerto Rican women had been diagnosed with mental illness. This higher proportion among the Puerto Rican women may have been due to our sampling procedures. Alternatively, the Puerto Rican participants may have had comparatively greater access to health care providers who, upon hearing and seeing their symptoms, formally assessed them for and diagnosed them with mental illness.

The higher prevalence of HIV risk behaviors among the women with severe mental illness perhaps should not have been so surprising. It has been estimated that almost one-third of the non-institutionalized U.S. population is affected by a diagnosable mental disorder each year, and almost one-half of the population is affected over the course of their lives.[5] And, since the identification of the first cases of AIDS in 1981, there has been a growing awareness of the increased risk of HIV infection associated with various mental illnesses. Researchers have consistently reported distressingly high prevalence rates of HIV infection and HIV risk behaviors among people with severe mental illness. Studies among sample populations with severe mental illness found that HIV seroprevalence ranged from 4 to 22.9 percent.[6] By contrast, the prevalence rate among the general population of the United States was 0.3 to 0.4 percent.[7] These studies indicate that HIV seroprevalence varies by age, gender, ethnicity, and treatment setting. Additionally, the prevalence of HIV among Hispanic people with severe mental illness has been found to be three times that among whites, suggesting that ethnicity "may play a role in the relative risk of exposure to HIV."[8]

These high rates of infection reflect the high prevalence of risk behaviors among individuals with severe mental illness. Although many researchers have assumed that adults with severe mental illness are not very active sexually,[9] as many as 40 percent of individuals with a severe mental illness report having had more than one sexual partner during the preceding year.[10] In fact, only 17 percent of the general U.S. population report having had more than one sexual partner during the year preceding their self-report.[11] As many as 20 to 26 percent of individuals with a severe mental illness report having had sexual intercourse with an injection drug user,[12] and as many as 27 percent or more have reported trading sex for drugs.[13] In one study of sixty adults with severe mental illness, 48 percent of the men and 37 percent of the women reported at least one HIV risk factor.[14] This high prevalence of HIV risk behaviors and HIV infection is particularly worrisome because many people with severe mental illness know relatively little about how HIV is transmitted or prevented and may rarely or inconsistently use condoms to reduce their risk of HIV infection.[15]

Women with severe mental illness may be at even greater risk of HIV infection. One study of 134 men and women with severe mental illness who reported having sexual activity outside an exclusive relationship or with high-risk partners found that *being female* predicted increased risk.[16] Women with mental illness may be at increased risk of HIV for a number of reasons. First, their mental illness may cause difficulty in processing information, so that they are less able to identify and avoid situations that are risky. Second, they may be less competent socially as a result of their illness, so that they are less able to form lasting relationships, refuse unreasonable requests, solve problems effectively, and negotiate risky situations.[17] Third, women with a severe mental illness may be at increased risk of partner violence,[18] which may place them at increased risk of HIV infection. Fourth, many of the women must struggle every day to survive in the face of poverty and unemployment; consequently, the risk of HIV infection and AIDS may not be a high priority in comparison to these other concerns.[19] Finally, as women, they are more vulnerable to HIV transmission because of the anatomical and hormonal differences that exist between men and women.[20]

Hispanic/Latino communities in the United States have also been disproportionately affected by HIV/AIDS. Although Latinos accounted for only 14 percent of the population, including Puerto Rico, in 2006 they accounted for 18 percent of all new HIV diagnoses reported in the thirty-three areas with long-term confidential name-based HIV reporting. As of 2006, they also accounted for 16 percent of all AIDS cases diagnosed since the beginning of the epidemic.[21] Recent reports indicate that the HIV prevalence rate for Hispanics is 585.3 individuals per 100,000 population, 2.6 times the rate for whites. Among Hispanic women, the prevalence rate is 263.0 per 100,000, more than four times the rate for non-Hispanic white women.[22] In 2004, an estimated 20.4 percent of all deaths attributed to AIDS were among Hispanics.[23] In 2002, HIV/AIDS became the fourth leading cause of death in the United States for Hispanics ages thirty-five to forty-four and the sixth leading cause of death among those ages forty-five to fifty-four. HIV disease now ranks as the third leading cause of death among Hispanic men ages thirty-five to forty-four and the fourth leading cause of death among Hispanic women of the same age group.[24] Puerto Ricans, in particular, have been disproportionately affected.[25]

In Cleveland, which is the largest city in northeastern Ohio, the site of this study, and which ranks as the thirty-ninth largest city in the United States, Hispanics account for 4 percent of the population. The HIV prevalence rate of 1,061.4 per 100,000 among Hispanics in Cleveland is higher than among any other racial/ethnic group. It is estimated that fully 1 percent of Cleveland's Hispanic population is HIV infected, compared to an estimated 0.6 percent prevalence within the general U.S. population.[26] Unprotected heterosexual intercourse remains the predominant mode of transmission for Puerto Rican women, both nationally and in Cuyahoga County. In Cleveland, 48 percent of all Hispanic females currently living with HIV/AIDS were infected through unprotected heterosexual intercourse, with the remainder having been infected through injection drug use, maternal transmission, and unknown routes.

These data prompted numerous questions for which we sought answers through the research that we describe in this volume. What is it about being female, about being a Latina, that results in an apparently increased risk for HIV? Is it attributable to relationship dynamics, or to factors within a larger socioeconomic-political context? Does the context of risk change depending on variations in diagnoses, Latino heritage, or geographic context?

A Word about Methodology

Eligibility for participation in this mixed methods study required a diagnosis of major depression, schizophrenia, or bipolar disorder and an age of between eighteen and fifty years at the time of enrollment. The study was initially designed to recruit seventy-five Puerto Rican women from the six-county area of northeastern Ohio and seventy-five women of Mexican ethnicity from San Diego County.[27] Each group of seventy-five was to consist of twenty-five women from each of the three diagnostic categories of interest.

We had anticipated that the recruitment of participants for the study would be challenging for any number of reasons. Individuals who acknowledge a diagnosis of severe mental illness are often stigmatized by family, friends, and their larger communities. It would be critical to develop a mechanism by which to communicate the focus of the study without requiring that individuals signal their status in front of others. Also, there existed the possibility of a significant power differential between our research team and our prospective participants because of wide differences in socioeconomic status and educational levels. The paranoia that is often characteristic of schizophrenia and bipolar disorder could also serve as a barrier to reaching and communicating with potentially eligible women. And, as in many other studies, it was likely that competing demands on time and financial resources could affect women's decision to participate in the study, particularly in view of the time commitment involved in shadowing and multiple interviews.

Accordingly, we developed an array of strategies to maximize recruitment and reassure potential participants that they would be safe and their concerns addressed (Table 1.1). We applied for a certificate of confidentiality from the NIH, which protected the data from discovery in civil and criminal proceedings.[28] We offered stipends to the women for their participation in the interviews, both to compensate them for any costs they might have incurred for transportation or child care and to thank them for their time. We scheduled interviews at times when it was most convenient for the individual participants, including evenings and weekends.

Perhaps most importantly and most unusually for academic-based research, our ethnographers, the individuals who would be responsible for presenting the study to diverse groups within the Puerto Rican and Mexican communities and for shadowing the women, were selected because their educational levels and life experiences were similar in some respects to those of many of our participants. Almost all of the women who were hired to work as ethnographers with the study had high school educations or the equivalent, but no college. They were all fluent in Spanish, and many had lived in the locales in which the participants had been born.

Table 1.1. Recruitment challenges and strategies

Challenge	Procedural/methodological strategies	Personnel strategies
Identifying potential participants	Establishment of Community Advisory Board Ethnographer outreach to community Identification of critical links	Selection of ethnographers Training of ethnographers
Distrust and fear	Presentations to community groups Recruitment at community sites Frequent contact with study team Detailed explanation of study	Selection of ethnographers Training of ethnographers Principal investigator and staff involvement with community
Level of psychopathology	Ethnographer outreach Ethnographer consistency Frequent contact with study team	Frequent contact with study team
Competing obligations	Ethnographer outreach Flexibility in scheduling and location	Staff commitment to flexibility Provision of child care
Financial considerations	Small incentive	
Stigma	Use of specific wording	Training of study team members

These similarities between the participants and the ethnographers would reduce the power differential, at least to some extent, and would increase both the participants' comfort level and the likelihood that the study team would be accepted in the communities. It was important, too, that ethnographers be familiar with the Latino community in which they would be working, in terms of the politics, the agency relationships, and the formal and informal channels of communication.

In some ways, this strategy was risky: if the ethnographers were too close to the women and their communities, they might be unable to detach emotionally in order to serve as observers. In fact, this was the case with two of our ethnographers, who left the project after finding that the issues they encountered while shadowing the study participants, such as partner violence, depression, and substance use, brought up unresolved issues from their own lives. We learned from this experience that success as an ethnographer with this study required not only an in-depth familiarity and some level of identification with the Latino community but also an ability to navigate outside of the Latino community and a vision of oneself as part of a larger community. Although our successful ethnographers were part of the Puerto Rican community, their cultural capital allowed them the opportunity to move beyond the microworld inhabited by our study participants. Accordingly, this ethnography is not in the tradition of Piri Thomas's *Down These Mean Streets* or Philippe Bourgois's *In Search of Respect: Selling Crack in El Barrio*, in which the ethnographer-author inhabits the same world as those who are participants in the research. I, the author, did not live in the same neighborhoods as our participants, although, unlike many principal investigators, I came to know the majority of our research participants and interact with them in their homes, bodegas, and churches.

Past research findings suggested that retention could present even greater challenges than initial recruitment. Less than 75 percent of mentally ill research participants may remain available for follow-up during the course of a longitudinal study.[29] Even lower retention rates have been reported among mentally ill individuals experiencing periods of homelessness. In one study of homeless, chronically mentally ill veterans, only 37.9 percent remained available for follow-up.[30] Accordingly, we developed intensive procedures designed to maximize retention that were integrated in some way into every contact with each participant.

Retention of participants was critical to the successful completion of the study because we intended to follow our participants for a two-year period. Our retention efforts were labor intensive (Table 1.2); only a few are detailed here. We used "anchoring strategies," obtaining contact information from each participant for three individuals who always knew her whereabouts and a release from her allowing us to contact each of them should we be unable to find her. These anchoring strategies would allow us to more easily track participants who became lost because of unstable living situations, homelessness, hospitalization or incarceration, and disrupted or violent relationships.[31] We updated this information at almost every interaction with either the participant or one of the listed contacts. Although other commentators have suggested that updating such information every two years is adequate to track study participants, we anticipated that our participants would move quite frequently and that if we updated this information at lengthier intervals, we would lose them for follow-up.[32] We sent numerous cards throughout the study to each participant, which served as a reminder about their role in the study but also provided us with up-to-date information from the post office about any relocation that might have occurred. We obtained each participant's consent to contact her health care providers and social service providers for the purpose of locating her if we were otherwise unable to do so. We awarded participants with culturally appropriate incentives to congratulate them as they completed increasing segments of shadowing time. As an example, we awarded T-shirts after the completion of all shadowing hours; the T-shirts bore the logo of the research study team, Comunidades Unidas para la Salud (Communities United for Health). We held an annual reception for participants, research collaborators, and agencies with which we interacted during the course of the study.

Prior to actually enrolling an individual as a participant in the study, we verified her mental illness diagnosis with the Structured Clinical Interview for Axis I DSM-IV Diagnoses (SCID). The SCID has been used with various populations in numerous countries, has been translated into Spanish, and has been found reliable and valid for use with Spanish-speaking patients.[33] Following this confirmation of the diagnosis and enrollment into the study, we conducted the baseline interview, which consisted of a semi-structured portion and various quantitative measures designed to assess substance use, acculturation, and HIV-related knowledge and behaviors. We supplemented and verified the quantitative results against the qualitative data that we gathered through the semi-structured part of the interviews and from the non-continuous participant observation. The structured instruments allowed us to standardize the informa-

Table 1.2. Retention strategies by study phase

Phase	Procedural/methodological strategy	Personnel strategy
Pre-recruitment	Community involvement in development of study protocol Community input into development of staff policies and procedures	Selection of study staff members Training of study team Development of staff policies and procedures manual Principal investigator interaction with relevant communities Formation of Community Advisory Board
Recruitment	Assistance from Community Advisory Board Provision of accurate and detailed information Emphasis on continuing nature of study Avoidance of stigmatizing labels Participant-centered approach Use of incentives	Training of study team
Enrollment	Anchoring strategies including obtaining —Contact information for participant —Contact information for key persons in participant's life —Contact information for participant's health care providers —Written consent from participant to contact individuals	Personnel training regarding informed consent process

Baseline interview	Participant provision of information about her usual hangouts Reminder about study protocol	Assignment to appropriate interviewer for follow-up
Follow-up	Updating of contact information for participant Updating of contact information for participant's contacts Small financial incentive Referrals for requested services Reminder about study procedures Holiday and birthday cards One-week reminders of appointments Twenty-four-hour reminders of appointments One-hour reminders of appointments Field and agency tracking Quarterly newsletters Annual reception Periodic congratulatory rewards Frequency and consistency of contact with designated staff Continuing interaction with Community Advisory Board	"Case" presentation/debriefing at team meetings Study team interaction with community Periodic re-training of study staff

tion we received and to provide a standard against which that information could be measured. Trained bilingual staff conducted all of the interviews and ethnographic observations.

As part of the baseline interview, we assessed the severity of each participant's substance use using the Addiction Severity Index (ASI). The ASI evaluates seven functional areas: medical status, employment and support, drug use, alcohol use, legal status, family/social status, and psychiatric status. We assessed acculturation using a short acculturation scale developed for use specifically with Latinos.[34] This assessment was important because lower levels of acculturation have been found to be associated with erroneous beliefs relating to HIV transmission, lower levels of HIV knowledge, greater reluctance to use condoms, lower levels of HIV disclosure to others, and risk behaviors for various other diseases.[35]

Since the level of HIV knowledge an individual possesses may be relevant to an understanding of the individual's behavior, we also assessed HIV knowledge and behaviors. This instrument included a twelve-item true-false scale designed to measure practical knowledge about HIV and risk behaviors in addition to items relating to condom efficacy, perceived risk, barriers to condom use, partner attitudes toward condom use, peer group use of condoms, barriers to HIV testing, barriers to clean needle use, and HIV prevention behaviors during the previous year. We had used this instrument previously in studies relating to HIV knowledge and attitudes and had found that it has excellent reliability.[36]

After the baseline interview, each participant was to be interviewed once a year for two years. We used ethnographic methods to "shadow" each participant for up to one hundred hours over a two-year period, observing them in various situations such as physician visits, hospital visits, appointments with mental health care providers, family events, church gatherings, parties, nightclubs, interactions with sexual or romantic partners and sexual clients, interactions with drug-using partners and while injecting, and interactions with children. Additionally, we conducted interviews each year for two years with a health care provider and a "critical other" designated by each participant. Our use of these varied methods of data collection and our reliance on multiple sources of data (Table 1.3) allowed us to triangulate the data—that is, to obtain data relating to the same topic from multiple sources of information—enabling us to verify the accuracy of information that came to us.

We tape-recorded most of the shadowing activities. However, in situations in which the safety of the participant, the ethnographer, or others

Table 1.3. Sources of data

Data	Source
Demographic information	Interviews Shadowing Medical records review
Language	Acculturation measure Interviews Shadowing
Mental illness diagnosis	Structured Clinical Interview (SCID) Medical records review
Substance use	Structured Clinical Interview (SCID) Addiction Severity Index (ASI) Self-report Shadowing Provider report Medical records review
Family composition and dynamics	Interview Critical-other interview Shadowing Provider report
Provider information	Interview Provider report Shadowing Medical records review
Medications prescribed	Interview Provider report Medical records review
Medication use	Interview Provider report Critical-other report Shadowing

could have been compromised, the ethnographer tape-recorded the observations she had had during the visit after she left the location of the shadowing. All tape recordings were transcribed in their original language; they were also translated into English if they were originally recorded in Spanish. We established a codebook, based both on predetermined themes noted in the previously published professional literature and on perspectives that arose from the data, and assigned codes on a line-by-line basis using Atlas.ti 5.0 software.[37] We created codes on a concurrent basis and assigned every paragraph in every transcription as many codes as was necessary to describe the contents of that paragraph accurately. This approach allowed for an examination of the data for patterns, themes, and categories developed by the participants.[38]

We used the data resulting from both our qualitative and quantitative approaches ("mixed methods") to understand the context in which our participants lived. Our mixed methods data-analysis process incorporated data reduction, display, transformation, correlation, consolidation, comparison, and integration.[39] In this study, data reduction involved exploratory thematic analysis of the qualitative data and descriptive analysis of the quantitative data. Data display involved describing the data pictorially using charts and networks for the qualitative data and tables and graphs for the quantitative data. We converted our qualitative data into numerical codes in order to represent the data statistically; that is, we *quantitized* the qualitative data.[40] The data correlation stage involved the correlation of qualitative data with any quantitized data. In the data consolidation stage, the quantitative and the qualitative data were combined to create new variables and a dataset for analyses. Finally, data comparison involved comparing data from the qualitative and quantitative data sources, and data integration provided a means to integrate the two types of data into a coherent whole.[41]

Approximately two years into the study, it became clear from the results of our preliminary data analysis that although our recruitment efforts at each site were highly successful, the same could not be said of our retention efforts. We had known that a proportion of our San Diego County participants were present in the United States illegally. Increased efforts by immigration authorities to detect, detain, and deport those believed to be in the country illegally affected not only those participants who were present illegally but even those who held a green card or a "mica," as the alien registration card signifying legal permanent residence is euphemistically called. As immigration officers began boarding buses, trains, and trolley cars and demanding the presentation of "papers" with increasing frequency, our participants became increasingly reluctant to venture outside of the immediate vicinity of their homes. Some modified their behavior to such an extent that they eliminated almost all contact with anyone other than their immediate family members. Many of these women had appeared to be more severely ill than their counterparts in Ohio, with less access to the medical care and supportive services that they needed in order to maintain a modicum of connection to what could be called objective reality. To some extent, their increased isolation may have been attributable to the severity of their illness, but some of the women clearly reduced their activities, such as frequenting nightclubs, in response to these intensified law enforcement efforts. We saw many of them move with increasing frequency in an attempt to evade detection. Some moved completely outside of the geographic areas of this study, and we were no longer able to locate them. Others were simply lost, presumably either having been discovered and deported or having gone so far underground that we could no longer locate them even through their known contacts, many of whom had also moved. These circumstances affected not only our ability to locate the women but also our ability to gain a clear understanding of their usual level of HIV risk.

In view of these circumstances, with the approval of our NIH program officer, we began recruiting women of Mexican ethnicity in the six-county area of northeastern Ohio, matching them by approximate age and diagnosis to the women recruited in San Diego. This allowed us to recruit and retain a greater number of Mexican women for the study than would have otherwise been possible. It also allowed us to determine whether the level of HIV risk among the women of Mexican ethnicity in northeastern Ohio was comparable to that of the Mexican women in San Diego.

It is not possible to completely understand the women's motivations for participating in this study. For some, the small periodic stipends of twenty dollars, which never totaled more than sixty dollars for any single participant, may have helped them to squeeze by during particularly difficult financial periods. For others, the ethnographer who followed them became a confidante who inhabited a world outside of their families and immediate circle, enabling the women to share their secrets in safety. For a small number of women, the similarities that they noted between themselves and the ethnographers in their style of dress, their hairstyles, and their makeup may have boosted their self-worth and self-esteem, providing validation of their value to themselves and to others. For still others,

Table 1.4. Demographic characteristics of the study participants (N = 53)

	Mean (SD)	Median (range)
Age in years at baseline	32.6 (8.7)	
Global Assessment of Functioning (GAF) score		60 (30–80)
Number of children		2 (0–7)
Education (number of years)		11 (6–16)

Characteristic		No.	%
Diagnosis	Bipolar disorder	19	35.8
	Major depression	28	52.8
	Schizophrenia	6	11.3
Baseline age in years	18–29	16	30.2
	30–39	21	40.0
	40–49	13	24.5
	50+	3	5.7
Education	Less than 12 years	28	52.9
	Completed high school	11	20.8
	Some college	14	26.4
Marital status	Never married	11	20.8
	Married/living with partner	35	66.0
	Divorced or separated	7	13.2
Number of children	None	5	9.4
	1–3	35	66.0
	4–8	13	24.5
Employment status	None	35	66.0
	Part-time	8	15.1
	Full-time	10	18.9
Primary source of income	SSI or other public source	28	52.8
	Employment	15	28.3
	Partner or other family member income	9	17.0
	Unknown	1	1.9
Place of birth	Mainland U.S.	12	22.6
	Puerto Rico	40	75.5
	Other country	1	1.9

continued

Table 1.4. *continued*

Characteristic		No.	%
Primary language	English	7	13.2
	Spanish	29	54.5
	English and Spanish equally	17	32.1
Religion at birth	Catholicism	40	75.5
	Pentecostal	9	17.0
	Protestantism (unspecified)	2	3.8
	Nonpracticing	1	1.9
	Unknown	1	1.9
Current religious practice	Catholicism	16	30.2
	Pentecostal	13	24.5
	Protestant (unspecified)	6	11.3
	Methodist	2	3.8
	Baptist	1	1.9
	Mita y Aron	1	1.9
	Pagan	1	1.9
	Nonpracticing	12	22.6
	Unknown	1	1.9

members of the study team became witnesses to their lives, validating the importance of their existence and ensuring through our writings that they would be remembered.

I focus here on the fifty-three Puerto Rican women of northeastern Ohio who participated in this study (Table 1.4). I have attempted to provide both our qualitative and quantitative findings and to place them in the context of existing research, in order to provide the reader with a more complete and textured understanding of the women and the settings in which they live. In some instances, I have included lengthy quotes, which allow the reader to hear the voices of the women themselves and to gain additional insight into the methodological underpinnings of the study. I have not included our findings relating to the Mexican women in this volume; the complexities of each group's situation and the vast differences that exist between the two groups of women preclude the possibility of adequately portraying each in the same volume.

I have altered the names of the individuals and the street locations of events in order to protect the women's privacy and safeguard their trust. I have also made every attempt to tell their story in their voice—hence the inclusion of excerpts in the original Spanish in which they were spoken—culled from thousands of hours of tape recordings that were transcribed verbatim and assiduously coded by multiple trained coders for analysis of themes and patterns.

The book is organized so that each chapter focuses on a specific aspect of the women's lives—mental illness, employment, relationships, family, and so forth. However, these various strands of the women's lives are intertwined; what occurs in one domain affects their situation in another. Poverty, mental illness, abuse—each individually increases the women's risk for substance use, for HIV, for yet additional victimization. I have attempted to point out the interconnections between these issues even while addressing a specific domain of the women's lives; life for them, as for all, is lived at the intersection of one's roles, responsibilities, statuses, and experiences.

2

Living with Mental Illness

No se que es lo que tengo.
[I don't know what it is that I have.]
—Yadra, speaking of her mental illness

Living with a mental illness is often fraught with difficulties and peril. First there is the period of time when a person doesn't know that she has a mental illness, but people around her wonder why she is behaving strangely, or maybe she knows that something is wrong but can't quite figure out what it is. So she goes to a doctor to find out what is bothering her, or is taken to the hospital because she tries to kill herself or threatens to kill someone else, and that is when she is told that she is mentally ill. Then comes that period of time when she must figure out what it all means. Maybe the person feels ashamed, wondering whether she has done something wrong and this is God's way of punishing her. She spends inordinate amounts of time trying to trace back in her life to the origin of the mysterious malady that she has been told is now hers for all time. She wonders whether she needs medication and whether she will be able to work. She also has to decide which of her family members and friends should be told, if any. "What will they say? What if they don't want me around anymore?" And, if she is feeling really bad, she might even ask, "Is someone going to take my kids away from me?"

Then, if the person has been able to get through all of this, she may face even more conundrums: "How do I keep from gaining weight with this medication?" "I live with my mother/sister/other relative because of my mental illness and she tells me what to do, but I have no choice if I want to live there." "What will happen to me when I die? Will God still want me?"

One or more of these questions plagued each of the fifty-three women who participated in this study. First, all of the women were faced with the task of what to name their illness. Second, the vast majority of the women spent large amounts of time sifting through the minute details of their lives in an attempt to understand the source of this named "thing" that seemed at times to exist separately from them, more than being a part of who they are. For some of the women, this meant trying to decipher the meanings underlying the label that had been conferred on them by a health care professional; other women attempted to understand why they behaved the way they did or why they felt the way they did. Finally, each of the women strived to understand the meaning of the illness and its impact, and to find ways of coping.

Naming "It"

Knowing one's diagnosis is not necessarily helpful. It is a label that is bestowed by a psychiatrist or psychologist or social worker and may have little or no relevance in the immediate context of one's life. In addition, when others learn of the label and respond to it, they often mistake it for the person, forcing the diagnostic label and its baggage into the foreground of that person's life. The categories that individuals use to describe their own illness, however, are immediately relevant because these

> illness categories can be understood as images which condense fields of experience, particularly of stressful experience. And they can be understood as core symbols in a semantic network, a network of words, situations, symptoms, and feelings which are associated with an illness and give it meaning for the sufferer. The meaning of an illness term is generated socially as it is used by individuals to articulate their experiences of conflict and stress, thus becoming linked to typical syndromes of stresses in the society.[1]

Thus, it was important for the women in our study to frame their own illness in a way that had meaning and was socially relevant to them and acceptable to those in their lives. It is similarly critical that we understand their perspective if we are to begin to fathom the complexity of their lives and their strategies for managing their realities.

Nervios

Many of the women referred to their illness as *nervios*, regardless of the formal medical diagnosis that they had received. Osana, for example, explained, "*Yo estoy mal de los nervios*" (literally, "I am sick from my nerves," signifying, "My nerves are bad"). By contrast, they referred to their symptoms as an *ataque de nervios*, literally "nervous attack" or "attack of the nerves."

The meaning and origin of these terms are significantly more complex than might be supposed from their translation. The women used the term *nervios* to refer to their underlying, long-term mental illness. Guarnaccia and colleagues explain,

> All forms of nervios are powerful idioms employed primarily by working class and poor Puerto Rican men and women to express personal distress, crises in the family, and social deprivation. . . . People recognize that many of life's lesions, such as family losses, abusive and violent family relationships, lack of economic resources, and the traumas of sending loved one's [*sic*] off to or going to war, can produce major alterations in one's nervios. . . . When one talks about one's nervios, one is talking as much about one's life circumstances and need for help as about bodily pains and emotional distress.[2]

By contrast, an *ataque* signifies a response to a specific traumatic event or experience and the unacceptability of one's situation.[3] A typical ataque may involve crying, screaming, fainting or falling-out spells, dizziness, shortness of breath, weakness, chest pain, or rapid breathing.[4] Symptoms of an ataque may occur in clusters: irritability and anger, nervousness and insecurity, sadness and depression, hopelessness and frustration or confusion.[5] The experience of an ataque communicates in a culturally and socially acceptable manner to others one's feeling that the world has gone out of control.[6]

Narcisa's report of the ataques that she suffered while she was hospitalized reflects this feeling that the world as she knew it was out of control. Narcisa had been diagnosed some time ago with bipolar disorder. As a child, she had been the victim of sexual abuse, and as an adult, she had survived the violent attacks of a romantic partner. Narcisa was confined to the psychiatric unit of a hospital because of her increased stress and depression and concern that she might try to harm herself like she had done on several occasions in the past:

> I had four attacks. *De los nervios.* [Of the nerves.] I had four attacks while I was hospitalized. I would call the nurses to tell them about the problems I was having but they did not care. I cursed and defended myself with the little bit of English that I could. . . . That place is crazy. They be having men and women in the same room. *A mi me vieron hasta desnuda.* [They even saw me naked.] Then they have people with mental problems in the same floor with other patients. That made me even more depressed. *Entre mala allí y salí peor.* [I went in there in bad shape and came out worse.] I had attacks because of my pressure. I was at first at [a local] hospital. I called [my counselor] because I was feeling a lot of pressure. She told me to go to the hospital. I have been under a lot of stress. [*Narcisa starts to cry.*] *Yo me siento mal. No puedo controlar esta depresión.* [I feel ill. I can't control my depression.]

By defining her experience as an ataque de nervios, Narcisa was able to draw a distinction between her identity and condition and those of her companions on the hospital floor who, because of their "mental problems," had been relegated to that "crazy" place. Her use of the term reflects her perception of and displeasure with her hospitalization, providing her with a mechanism by which she may distance herself from those whom she perceives as truly ill and beyond either hope or help.

The term *ataques de nervios* has frequently been misunderstood within the medical profession. The term was first used in the medical literature in 1955 to describe what was perceived by U.S. Army psychiatrists as extreme emotional reactions among Puerto Rican army recruits. Not understanding the significance or meaning of these symptoms, they pathologized the common phenomenon of ataques by fashioning a new and pejorative diagnostic category: the Puerto Rican syndrome, or PRS.[7] More insightful scholars have asserted that this label reflects the power relationship that existed between the army psychiatrists and the Puerto Rican inductees at a specific location during a specific point in time.[8] It also serves to create and reinforce differentness and the conceptualization of the Other:

> The Puerto Rican syndrome presents itself as a riddle. The riddle supposes an other (an Army doctor, an espiritista, a social worker, a psychoanalyst) capable of solving it. This enigmatic set of symptoms

> compels this other to respond: as if asking the question "What am I?" or better said, "Tell me who I am so that I can know what you want me to be." These questions ask, in fact: "What am I for the Other?" This is a question that asks for an answer that is doomed to fail, because no answer can make things whole.[9]

The occurrence of ataques is not unique to the women who participated in this study, but is a relatively frequent expression of emotional distress among Puerto Ricans. It has been estimated that 14 percent of Puerto Rico's inhabitants experience an ataque at some point in their lives, while up to 75 percent of mental health patients have reported experiencing at least one ataque.[10] Although ataques de nervios have been associated with the diagnostic criteria for a variety of anxiety, affective, and panic disorders,[11] an ataque may occur in the absence of any pathology and is perceived as a normal and expectable response.[12] Modern-day psychiatry, however, views an ataque de nervios as a "culture-bound syndrome," essentially pathologizing "ordinary and extraordinary experience and [disaffirming] the meaning-oriented subjectivity of suffering in favor of technical diagnoses that often lack personal and collective significance."[13] The characterization of an ataque as "culture-bound" necessarily implies that U.S. culture and psychiatric dogma are the standard against which the normality of responses are to be judged; to be "culture-bound" is to be the "Other."[14]

Being Crazy, Loca

A few of the women referred to themselves as crazy, *loca*. Katia, for instance, who had been diagnosed with bipolar disorder, explained that we had been unable to locate her the previous week because she had been "*loca otra vez*" (crazy again) and "tried to commit suicide again." Because of her craziness, she confided, she had been confined involuntarily to the psychiatric unit of a local hospital.

Maria suffered from depression and had frequent auditory and visual hallucinations. She often referred to her head as "a crazy computer," wiping her eyes as she cried, "Yep, that is how schizophrenia is, a lot of hallucinations. I was confused." Honoria also understood the severity of her own illness. Twenty-eight years old at the time she entered the study, Honoria had been diagnosed with bipolar disorder. Her conversations with our ethnographer Isa were directed as much toward her cat as they were toward Isa. Despondent and frustrated by her own illness, she lamented to both Isa and her cat, "I want to go to the hospital and be locked up. . . . I feel like I can't control myself."

In one sense, Katia's and Maria's characterization of their conditions as "crazy" and Honoria's recognition of her need for hospitalization reflect a greater level of insight into the nature and severity of their illness, compared to the awareness of many of the other women. One could argue that this greater insight into their illnesses would serve them well by allowing them to take positive steps toward the amelioration of symptoms. In another sense, however, their characterization of themselves as "crazy" and their recognition of the severity of their illnesses signal their resignation to their situations.

Understanding the Source

Modern-day psychiatry often views diseases such as schizophrenia, bipolar disorder, and depression as entities with a biological or genetic basis[15] that require pharmacotherapy and perhaps psychoeducation and some form of verbal or other therapy to augment the use of medication.[16] Similar to findings of other researchers, we found that many of the women in our study rejected medical or biological explanations for their illness in favor of environment-based interpretations.[17]

Mental illnesses have been linked to a variety of social and environmental circumstances, including obstetric complications, poverty, and urbanicity.[18] Trauma such as childhood sexual and physical abuse,[19] and intrafamilial childhood sexual abuse in particular,[20] has been linked to the later development of multiple major psychiatric disorders. It has been hypothesized that posttraumatic stress disorder (PTSD) may lead to severe mental illness, either directly or indirectly. PTSD may affect psychosis directly through the effects of specific PTSD symptoms, such as avoidance and re-experiencing the original trauma. Indirect effects may operate through the consequences of PTSD, such as retraumatization in the context of new experiences, interpersonal difficulties, and substance abuse. It has also been suggested that the traumatic experiences may lead to the development of faulty self and social knowledge and affect the individual's interpretations of events,[21] and that dissociative symptoms resulting from the initial traumatic experience may place an individual at increased risk of psychosis.[22] Data suggest that both sexual abuse and physical abuse are surprisingly common childhood experiences, respectively affecting 32.3 percent and 19.5 percent of female children.[23] However, many of these individuals develop trauma-related symptoms but do not develop psychiatric disorders in later life. The precise mechanism of the association between abuse and severe mental illness remains unclear.

Witnessing Violence

Yadra struggled to understand why she was depressed, why she continually had thoughts of harming herself. She attributed her lack of energy, her fears, and her difficulties dealing with life's daily tribulations to an earlier, horrifying experience:

> I was fifteen years old. It was in my house in Puerto Rico after Hurricane Hugo had passed. It was dark because there was no electricity. Two guys passed by and asked for a glass of water. They entered my living room and sat down. One of the guys was my husband's brother. I went to get the water, and two other guys walked in and shot the guys in the living room in the head. *Los cesos estaban en mi camisa.* [Their brains were all on my shirt.] When I went to the burial it was awful because the family members of the two guys killed blamed me because it happened in my house. After the age of seventeen was when it really started affecting me. Since then I have flashbacks of what happened. I relive the events from the time I went to get the water till the time where they got killed. The killers were never found. *No tengo vida social. El trauma mío de los asesinatos me daño la vida.* [I don't have a social life. My trauma from the murders ruined my life.]

Several participants remembered first feeling their symptoms of depression following a terrible incident with their children. Pia, who had tried to kill herself several times, recounted, "I started feeling that way back in the '90s when my son was nine years old. He was hit by a car and went into a coma for fifteen days. I was in recovery for four months." Laurita's young son had died in a terrible house fire that had been set by some older children in the neighborhood. During an appointment with her physician, she explained the impact of his death on her:

> I have nightmares of my son dying in the fire. It was a while back. . . . He was eight months old, he died in front of my eyes. [*Laurita is shaking and tears stream down her cheeks.*] He died in a fire. I have dreams of his stomach being open and his body stuffed with cotton. I dream of him getting dressed in the funeral home and turning his head only to see the stitches around his head. It was my son. I took pills two or three months ago. I wanted to sleep. . . . It was 1993 [nine years ago]. Someone rescued me. Kids set the house on fire. It was my fault. It was my responsibility to save him. It was my child. I am slow in doing things. I want to be with my kids, the world is dead for me. I had a son, I had a job.

Experiencing Violence

Many of the women traced their first experience of their symptoms, their first feelings that something was different for them and about them, to their abuse as children. Narcisa, for example, explained how the sexual abuse that she had suffered as a child continued to haunt her even as an adult:

> I had such awful experiences. When I was little, my grandfather used to touch me in my private parts and he would try to penetrate me but I would tighten my legs. I thank God that he was never able to. I finally told my grandmother and she kicked me out of the house. She told me to get my stuff and get out. . . . Since the age of five, I remember my grandfather, my dad, and my uncle removing my underwears [*sic*] and touching me. *Yo tengo como un trauma que no se me quede quitar. No es facil.* [I have, like, a trauma that does not go away. It is not easy.]

What Narcisa didn't know, and perhaps would never understand because of the impaired judgment that resulted from her mental illness, was that her traumatic sexual experiences might be tied in some way to her current sexual activities, her romantic involvement with men who abused her, and her level of HIV risk. (The relationship between sexual trauma and HIV risk is explored further in Chapter 8.)

Teodora, too, believed that her illness resulted from the multiple episodes of sexual abuse that she had endured:

> When I was fourteen years old I went to the mental hospital. I went twice to the mental hospital. One time for two and a half years. That time I was twelve years old. I was raped when I was five years old by [my brothers] Roberto, Andres, and my father. I never said nothing until I was seven. It's like a Lifetime movie.[24] It got to the point I started hallucinating of [my father]. Yeah, they had to strap me down in the hospital.

Her mental health care providers tried to dissuade Teodora from attributing her illness to this abuse by carefully explaining the biological basis for bipolar disorder and pointing to her family history of mental illness, believing that this information might increase the likelihood that Teodora would use the medication prescribed for her. Teodora readily acknowledged her family history, describing her family as "a Jerry Springer family: My grandma had depression and my uncle uses alcohol and drugs. My grandpa is an alcoholic. My aunts do coke and crack, O and X. You guys know Delfina, she is coked out. . . . My dad has mental problems. Roberto has borderline personality disorder and Andres is bipolar, both of my brothers are mental cases."[25]

Like Teodora, Lalia, a forty-three-year-old woman who had been diagnosed with schizophrenia, did not believe her psychiatrist's explanation about the biological basis of her mental illness. Rather, she believed that her illness had been brought about by a burn that occurred when she was quite young. She mused,

> I know that my condition was not something I inherited. I developed this condition because of a burn I suffered when I was three years old. Well, I was three years old and I was really sick with a fever. My mom bathed me with alcohol and *alcolado* [a mixture of herbs and alcohol]. My hair was soaked in it. My brother Teodor was playing with a toy gun that sparked. He did it next to me and my hair lit up in fire, and it burned the whole side of my face. I was six years without being able to grow hair. That is why my brother Tito and I are so close, 'cause he always felt terrible about that incident. I remember I had a blue bed with a *mosquitero* [mosquito net] on it because of my burn. I remember that there were always two angels with me in that crib. One was black and the other white. The white angel was always really nice and playful with me. The black one would bother me. He would tickle my feet and pull my toes.

> At that time there were no surgeons like we have now. At the age of fifteen surgery was not recommended to repair the damages to my face. Then they started inserting cortisone into my face. That was hell. But even though I had defects on my face I still won several beauty contests in Puerto Rico. But I have always been insecure about the scars on face. I am going next month to see a surgeon . . . to see what he says. My mom took me to a psychiatrist at the age of nine. The doctor said that the burn affected my nervous system. Throughout my adolescent years I had a hard time accepting the imperfections of my face but like I told you I was still a professional model. I was a beauty queen two times. What I think it has affected the most is my learning and the trouble I have with my memory. *Siempre fui una muchacha tranquila.* [I was always a calm girl.] I always got extra attention from my mom, brothers, and sisters, but I think that was just because of my personality and not my condition.

Our research team never knew whether Lalia had in fact suffered such severe burns, or any burns, for that matter. We never saw any scars, even on those occasions when she did not wear makeup. The burns might have healed over time, but because Lalia had never had plastic surgery, it seemed unlikely that such severe burns could have healed so thoroughly by early adolescence that she could have won a beauty pageant. Lalia often confused dates and times and even how many children she had had. If Lalia had indeed suffered these burns, and if her doctor had indicated that the burns had affected her nervous system, Lalia may have interpreted the statement quite differently than how it was intended. Whereas the doctor may have been referring to injury to Lalia's physical nerves as a result of the burn, Lalia had surmised that the damage was to her emotional state, her nervios.

Other Causes

Less frequently, participants attributed their illness to magic, a curse, or witchcraft. Cassandra, for example, adhered to *Espiritismo*, a form of indigenous therapy that is believed to provide an outlet for frustration and aggression, permit catharsis, and provide a "corrective emotional experience."[26] Consistent with her spiritual beliefs, Cassandra felt that both the termination of her romantic relationship and the concurrent onset of her mental illness resulted from a curse that had been placed on her by her beloved's mother: "We broke up because of his mother. His mother was a *bruja* [witch]. She didn't want him to be with me. She didn't think I would make her son happy. She did witchcraft and she put a spell on me." Cassandra planned to seek revenge through another bruja, who would be able to use witchcraft to cast spells and call upon spirits to work against her boyfriend's mother. Additionally, an *espiritista*, or medium, could prescribe behaviors, tasks, or rituals that the affected individual could use to eliminate or overcome the spell.[27]

Adalia, too, believed that her depression resulted from a curse, as she explained to Isa, one of the study ethnographers:

> ADALIA: I went to a psychic and he told me someone put a curse on me with an illness [depression]. . . . Yes, he said they put in me an illness. . . . Well, it can happen because they don't get along with me and the psychic told me.
>
> ISA: Who's the psychic?
>
> ADALIA: *Un señor* [a man].

Adalia believed that the psychic had the power to cure her. She recounted the healing episode that she had with him: "He cleaned [cured] me with a coconut and the coconut broke. When the coconut breaks the illness goes away. Let me see, this happened a week ago. My mother even knows him. I told him I had faith I was going to be healed." Despite her faith in this process, Adalia's depression remained uncured and she remained on medication for her depression.

Keeping It Together—or Not

Self-Isolation

Many of the women who had experienced or witnessed a traumatic event isolated themselves from others in an attempt to avoid any possible threat of witnessing or experiencing yet another horror. Yadra, who had been covered with the brains and blood of the men whose murders she witnessed, explained,

> My nerves don't let me go out. . . . I am afraid that I will witness a crime of someone being killed in front of me like I did before. *Si esta en mi encerrarme en esta casa para que nadie me humille yo lo hago. Mi vida no vale nada. Mi vida es mierda. Tu te crees que esto es vida, estar encerrada en la casa? Esto no es vida.* [If it is in me to lock myself up in this house so no one could humiliate me, I would do it. My life has no worth. My life is shit. Do you think this is life to be locked up in the house? This is not life.]

The events of the killings continued to haunt Yadra, even decades after their occurrence, despite counseling and medication: "*Todo me sale mal. Yo no dormí llorando y pidiendole a Dios que me quite esas cosas de la mente. Pienso en como matarme.*" (Everything comes out wrong. And I can't sleep, crying and begging God to take these things out of my head. I think about how to kill myself.) Yadra frequently contemplated suicide, believing that it was the only resolution to her continual distress: "*No se ya que hacer. Muchas cosas en mi mente. El unico escape es lo que te digo. Así no tengo que resolver los problemas de nadie.*" (I don't know anymore what to do. A lot of things on my mind. The only escape is what I told you [suicide]. That way I don't have to solve everyone else's problems.) Yadra searched for meaning to her life, alternately blaming herself and the trauma of the killings for her difficulties: "*Algo tiene Dios para mi.* [God has something for me.] I was the one that destroyed my life. I am here for my kids. I dedicate myself to them. So I have meaning to live."

Katia, like Yadra, wanted others to leave her in peace. Katia was thirty-three at the time she joined the study. She had been sexually abused, and her current steady boyfriend often used her as an emotional and physical punching bag. Like many of the other study participants who had been diagnosed with bipolar disorder, Katia had a history of extensive drug use; in her case, she had used marijuana, crack, cocaine, and LSD (acid) in the past (Table 2.1).

Katia was also a cutter, frequently using a knife to make small incisions on her arm, watching the blood slowly flow out, in an attempt to make herself feel anything in those moments when she could not and to punish herself during those moments when her self-hatred was more than she could bear. Although we could not be sure, it may have also been Katia's replacement for suicide, which she had attempted several times in the past, or perhaps her expression of family dysfunction. Cutting is much

Table 2.1. Illness characteristics of the study participants (N = 53)

	Characteristic	No.	%	p-value[a]
Global Assessment of Functioning (GAF) score	30–40	4	7.6	
	41–50	12	22.6	
	51–60	12	22.6	
	61–70	16	30.2	
	71+	9	17.0	0.47
Diagnosis	Bipolar disorder	19	35.9	
	Major depression	28	52.8	
	Schizophrenia	6	11.3	0.27
Hallucinations	None	37	69.8	
	Visual	3	5.7	
	Auditory	10	18.9	
	Visual and auditory	3	5.7	0.76
Suicidal ideation	None	7	13.2	
	Past only	20	37.7	
	Current only	3	5.7	
	Past and current	23	43.4	0.67
Suicide attempts	Never	22	41.5	
	One	13	24.5	
	More than one	18	34.0	0.68
Self-injurious behaviors	None	44	83.0	
	Cutting	7	13.2	
	Bingeing or purging	1	1.9	
	Burning	1	1.9	0.96
Lifetime substance use	None	13	24.5	
	Alcohol only	7	13.2	
	Illegal drug only	3	5.7	
	Alcohol and illegal drug	28	52.8	
	Unknown	2	3.8	0.07
Current substance use	None	24	45.3	
	Alcohol only	10	18.9	
	Illegal drug only	3	5.7	
	Alcohol and illegal drug	14	26.4	
	Unknown	2	3.8	0.00

a. *p*-value is for Fisher's exact test

more common than one might think; 1,800 per 100,000 adolescents and young adults between the ages of fifteen and thirty-three engage in some form of self-mutilation, including cutting.[28] Katia's frequent cutting may have been related both to her unresolved conflicts around sexuality and menarche and to her high level of sexual risk behaviors.[29]

Katia had developed a reputation for being crazy, losing her temper, and becoming violent with others. Even her boyfriend, she reported, was "scared" of her sometimes. Katia explained how she used her reputation as crazy and violent to her own benefit: "It's best for people to think I'm crazy. Because when people think you are crazy they leave you alone and don't bother you."

Lalia also tried to keep people away from her, for fear that they will be able to detect her mental illness. She explained,

> *A mi no me gusta que me visiten. No me gusta tener amigas.* [I don't like for people to visit me. I do not like having friends.] I don't like being around people because I am scared that they will be able to tell that I have a nervous condition. *La gente me lo notan y yo no se porque. Se me nota.* [People notice, and I do not know how. You can tell.] Maybe my hand expressions and the fact that I bite my nails gives it away or the fact that I don't want to talk. People come up to me and ask me if I have a nervous condition. It makes me angry, and I just walk away upset.

Substance Use and Abuse

At the time of the study, 51 percent of the women reported current use of alcohol or other substances (see Table 2.1). The frequency of their use ranged from rare use to daily consumption, and the quantity of their use varied just as widely. In addition, 71.7 percent of the women reported ever using any substance, including alcohol, over the course of their lifetime, and almost one-quarter of them (24.5 percent) had been diagnosed with substance abuse or dependence. These self-reports are consistent with what we know about the use of substances among individuals with a severe mental illness; up to half of all individuals with severe mental illness may develop substance abuse or dependence at some point during their lives.[30] Additionally, it has been estimated that 14.5 percent of individuals with bipolar disorder, 10.1 percent of those with schizophrenia, and 4.1 percent of those suffering from major depression also abuse substances.[31]

Scholars have argued that individuals with severe mental illness may turn to substances in an effort to relieve the symptoms of their mental illness that are not adequately controlled by medication, to reduce the uncomfortable side effects of their medication, to experience emotions when they are absent, or to help control emotions when they are confusing.[32] In fact, there is some research evidence to suggest that, at least for a proportion of individuals with psychiatric diagnoses, some substance use may indeed ameliorate various symptoms of their illness.[33] Katia explained how marijuana helped her to control her moods and how cocaine exacerbated her paranoia: "I like to smoke my weed. . . . It mellows me out. I used to drink a lot up to four days in a row. I sniffed a lot too but now I just smoke weed. Weed calms me down so I won't get into shit. Coke gets your teeth all fucked up and I used to get paranoid when I did coke."

Hermosa, too, used drugs to help her remain calm and relieve her depression. When we first recruited Hermosa to join the study, she had been sober and abstinent from drugs for over a year, successfully abstaining from using what had been her drugs of choice: alcohol, crack cocaine, and heroin. In the early days of our shadowing with Hermosa, during the time when she was abstinent from drugs, she eagerly greeted our ethnographer Isa at each visit, often running down the stairs from her second floor apartment to meet her in the large entryway of her apartment building. Hermosa took care with her appearance. In those days, she often sported large hoop earrings and multiple long gold chains. Her bright red and yellow clothing matched her buoyant mood. Hermosa had furnished her small apartment, consisting of a dining room, a kitchen, a bathroom, and a living room that doubled as her bedroom, quite stylishly and comfortably.

Hermosa was struggling to re-establish a reputation in her community as a *mujer buena*, a good woman, to recover from her prevailing image as a "heroin whore." Before she got off drugs, she had even had an affair (or she fantasized about having had an affair—we were never really sure which) with a married preacher, who she said had told her that the affair wasn't sinful and that a condom wasn't necessary because he was a man of God. The situation seemed to have at least a partial basis in objective reality, as she recounted how the once-friendly minister's wife suddenly distanced herself from Hermosa and other parishioners began to shun her.

Over time, we saw Hermosa become increasingly depressed and her tiny apartment increasingly devoid of accoutrements as she resumed her drug use. Gradually, she parted with the gold chains that she had prized, selling them and her furniture in an effort to pay off her mounting drug debts. Hermosa explained, somewhat disjointedly, why she had been unable to see us one day:

> *Ese día yo estaba deprimida no te voy a negar y me bebí un paquete de cerveza porque la depresión era mucho y mas cuando sentí que quería hablarme confundí me mente otra vez, yo me fui compre un paquete de cerveza.* [That day I was depressed and I refused to see you and I drank a six-pack of beer because the depression was too much and more when I felt that I wanted to talk I was confused again, and I went to buy a six-pack of beer.]

On another occasion, as she reached for a beer, Hermosa remarked, "Beer calms me down, so that is why I am drinking." Whether her shaking during that visit was due to her uncontrolled emotions, withdrawal from alcohol, withdrawal from heroin, or any combination of these possibilities was never entirely clear. The ethnographer noted in her personal observations of this shadowing: "This visit was hard to document because Hermosa's speech was slurred. Her eyes were red, and I smelled the alcohol on her. She moved around a lot and repeated things a lot. During this visit Hermosa told us she was now smoking crack everyday. . . . Hermosa disclosed that all the neighbors were using drugs and some were selling. . . . Hermosa now is asking us for money."

Why an individual uses a particular substance may depend on any number of factors, such as the cost and availability of a particular substance, the individual's income, the effort involved in obtaining and sustaining the use of a particular substance, and the degree to which others in the individual's network are also using that substance.[34] (The importance of individuals' social network is explored more fully in Chapter 5.) Wera, for example, recognized how difficult it is for someone to stop using when their friends and family are using. She explained to the ethnographer, Juanita, why her boyfriend was unlikely to stop using heroin:

> JUANITA: What is Agustin's drug of choice?
>
> WERA: *Yo no se por que el no hace esas porquerias al frente de mi. Creo que es la heroína y la usa por la nariz. Yo se que a el le gustaría dejarla pero*

yo quiero que lo haga ya, mañana. [I don't even know because he does not do that junk in front of me. I think it's heroin and he uses it through the nose. I know that he would like to leave it but I want him to do it now, tomorrow.]

JUANITA: I hear heroin is a hard drug to overcome. Do you think he would have support from his family if he tried to quit?

WERA: It would be really hard because almost his entire family uses. Out of that family, the only ones that do not use is the mom and two of the sisters. The mom had about five or six kids and they all use. When Agustin was a youngster he only smoked weed once in a while. On one of his birthdays his brother had him try heroin. *Desde eso esta huckiao.* [Ever since that he has been hooked.] From his own brother.

Hermosa, too, despite having had a year of sobriety and abstinence from drugs when we first met her, had begun using again during the course of the study when her new boyfriend turned to heroin and encouraged her to use the drug with him. Relapse is common, though, among individuals trying to rid themselves of drug addiction and is likely due, at least in part, to a deficit or sensitization in the brain's neurochemical reward system.[35] Crying, Hermosa said, "He was the one who gave it to me. . . . I thought nothing would happen and I would be clean in the morning. I am going to die soon. I am using and have liver problems . . . one bag of heroin a day and one pipoma [forty ounces of beer]."

Katia expressed concern about her daughter Kara and her use of drugs, knowing the crowd that she hung out with:

KATIA: I'm worried about Kara.

ISA: Why?

KATIA: She doesn't like to listen. Kara will try anything.

ISA: Like what?

KATIA: Like drugs and everything. She is a follower and I know she'll try anything.

Some of the women had begun using drugs as a way of making it through tough days and avoiding painful emotions.[36] In some cases, it's difficult to know whether their drug use began first and led somehow to their mental illness, or whether the symptoms of their mental illness affected their ability to deal with life's extraordinary difficulties, so that drugs provided a welcome escape from seemingly unending pain. Elena, for example, traced the beginnings of her relationship with alcohol to her parents' separation when she was just beginning to enter adolescence:

> I used to drink every day. I used to go to the bars and drank a lot of rum. I drank with my friends since I was thirteen years old. My mother noticed when I was eighteen years old. I went crazy when I turned twenty-one years old, started drinking a lot of beer. I didn't pay her rent because I spent money all on alcohol. . . . Back then I could not cut back and I drank a twelve-pack a day for twenty years. I went to work drunk and did not eat so I lost weight.

We do not know, and Elena could not remember, whether she had begun to experience any of the symptoms of what she now knows is schizophrenia, such as the voices commanding her to kill herself, prior to the time she began drinking. Nevertheless, Elena told Isa during a shadowing visit at her home, "I always knew there was something wrong."

Katia, too, traced the beginnings of her drug use to emotional pain—in this case, related to her mother's relinquishment of her after her mother's boyfriend tried to kill her. Rather than losing her boyfriend, her mother simply gave her up. Katia recounted, crying, "What messed me up is my mom giving me away. She doesn't love me. I love her. . . . Yes, she gave me away 'cause of her boyfriend. He wanted to kill me. . . . I went to the streets and started using drugs."

Katia's mental health care provider intimated that by the age of thirty-three, an adult woman would have or should have been able to somehow get beyond the pain of abandonment. But Katia had been dealt multiple burdens from the time she was born, and these burdens seemed to be ever-increasing, sometimes through her own purposeful actions, sometimes as a result of emotional outbursts that seemed to be beyond her control, and sometimes as a result of events truly beyond her control.

Regardless of why some of the women turned to drugs or alcohol, those who did often placed themselves further in harm's way, however unknowing they may have been. Their use of drugs and alcohol likely left them even more vulnerable to violence and to HIV than they might have been because of their mental illness alone. (These issues are discussed in greater detail in Chapters 4 and 8.)

Some of the women knew better than to use drugs as a way out, realizing that drugs would only worsen their situation. Laurita, for example, made her opinion about heroin use known in a comment to one of the ethnographers about a friend of her then-current partner:

> LAURITA: Ricardo has a friend that comes over. He injects drugs and I don't like that stuff.
> JUANITA: What do you think about it?
> LAURITA: It's stupid. You are never in reality. You are eating your brains out.

Maria, who had been diagnosed with schizophrenia, had previously abused alcohol, drinking from eight a.m. every day until she passed out from the alcohol at five p.m. When she would run out of alcohol late at night and no stores were open, she would drink isopropyl rubbing alcohol instead. The alcohol, she said, helped to obliterate the nightmares that she often experienced of worms crawling out of her arms and snakes and roaches crawling on her body; she did not seem to understand that these images may have resulted from her withdrawal from alcohol during the periods when she had none. Looking back at herself, Maria commented, "*Eso estaba cabron.*" (That was fucked up.) Maria told us that she had come to recognize that getting drunk had often led to her getting into trouble by starting physical fights with other people:

> Beer would not give me a buzz so I started to drink rum. It made me feel buzzed and good. Rum would really get me drunk. . . . I used to finish the night off . . . drinking Malibu and by this time I was ready to fight. When I used to drink, I thought I was Superwoman and wanted to kick everyone's ass. *Yo era loca; al quien se me metia en la cara le raspada una bofetada.* [I was crazy; whoever was in my face, I slapped them.]

Maria claimed to have forsworn alcohol forever more. We weren't sure how accurate her report was of having stopped drinking completely, however, because we knew that she still partied on a regular basis on Saturday nights, frequenting nightclubs with her friends. One Saturday night, our ethnographer Isa joined Maria at her favorite nightclub for shadowing. Maria had dressed for the occasion, sporting makeup, black spandex pants with a striped beige and black shirt, black sandals, and white fake-pearl earrings. Maria caught Isa eyeing the three bottles of beer and other mixed drinks on the table where she was sitting with her friend and quickly interjected, "I have juice. . . . The first year is the hardest to stop drinking. I can't ever drink again." Now, instead of drinking, Maria tried to find strength through the angels and saints and Virgin Marys that she bought for protection from the local thrift store for the various rooms of her small apartment and her collection of books from Alcoholics Anonymous that filled her bookshelf.

Finding Strength

Despite the many traumatic events and disappointments that they had experienced as children and as adults, the vast majority of the women had been able to identify and hold on to a variety of sources of strength. Fully 20 percent of our participants reported that they relied on religious or spiritual beliefs and rituals. This is not surprising in view of the important role that religion plays in the lives of many Hispanics.[37] In addition, many severely mentally ill individuals rely on religion as a source of hope, comfort, love, acceptance, and strength;[38] as a means of coping; and as a provider of role models for behavior, socialization opportunities, and material assistance, such as food and clothing.[39]

More than two-thirds of the women identified themselves as adherents to a specific faith community, although a substantial proportion had changed their religious affiliation from that of their upbringing. Of the forty women who had been raised in the Catholic faith, nine (22.5 percent) indicated that they had left the church and were now affiliated with another denomination, while an additional eight (20 percent) had ceased practicing any religion. Two women who had not been raised with a specifically identified religion had begun practicing Catholicism. Thirteen women self-identified as believers of the Pentecostal faith, although only nine had been raised in that faith. These realignments of faith mirrored the religious and spiritual trends that have been noted among Puerto Ricans in more recent years. Although Catholicism has played a major role in the lives of Puerto Ricans in Puerto Rico and on the U.S. mainland, a number of evangelical Protestant sects have experienced a dramatic increase in the number of Puerto Rican adherents, and more than one-third of all Puerto Ricans now self-identify as Protestant. In addition, many Puerto Ricans may practice Catholicism, Santeria, and Espiritismo simultaneously.[40]

During difficult times, a number of the women turned to God for support as they struggled to make their way through a seemingly endless abyss. Vyna wrote in her diary, "I run and run but I don't know where I'm going. I come to a stop. Why, I have no idea. All I know is that I'm scared. I ask that you help my soul find a place to stay warm, and keep it there. My God, what has happened to me?! I can't find a way out of this world of mine. Help me God."

Many of the women did find strength in their faith to help them manage the symptoms of their mental illness. Mila explained why she believed so many people have problems in life and how her life had changed since she had found Christ:

> I think that young people turn to drugs to make themselves feel better and to try and escape from reality. We were talking about this at Sunday school. It's the same thing with alcoholics. They can't handle their problems and then they lead to the bigger problem of addiction. *Tenemos que dejar el mundo.* [We need to leave the world.] That includes dancing, drinking, and smoking. . . . There are things like we cannot cut or dye our hair. We can't take out our eyebrows. I mean you can do it to a minimum but not too extravagant. Once you are faithful to the church you must be able to fight evil and maintain. People need to live in the evangelism. If you have lived it and left it your punishment will be seven times worse. *Todo lo que dice la biblia se cumple.* [Everything that the Bible says happens.] It's in the Bible. Before I was in the church I was a different person but I repented for the things I had done and gave my life to Christ.

Osana attributed her more recent improved mental outlook to the influence of God in her life:

> I don't want to get like I was before. I panic all the time. *Le tenia miedo a la noche porque otro dia venia. Yo era mala, yo robe por drogas. Pero, una cosa te digo, yo nunca perdí mi fe.* [I was scared of the night because another day was coming. I used to be bad, I stole for drugs. But one thing, I tell you, I never lost was my faith.] . . . I put up with a lot of things. . . . Now, I feel peaceful because of God.

Maria also found peace and relief from worry through her belief in God:

> God tells you not to worry about tomorrow because tomorrow is not promised. The birds don't have any clothes but God provides. We are

his children and he will provide. Sometimes we feel sad because we are human, but you ask God and you will feel better. Worrying affects your mind. How many thoughts race through your mind during the day![41]

Many women valued the compassion that they received from clergy, the families of clergy, and other church members. Hermosa reminisced about the sympathy that she had received from the minister's wife. Although Hermosa had not appreciated it at the time that it had been offered, she remembered the exchange wistfully:

> *Si, yo enferma de la droga. Y ella mudándome mis mattress y mis mesas. Y yo la veía y me daba una compasión pero a la misma ves estaba en el vicio so no me importaba, entiendes, no me importaba. No tenía el temor de dios que tengo ahora. Yo a hecho tantas tantas que yo a veces pienso que Dios no me va a perdonar lo que yo a hecho.* [Yes, I was sick with the drug (heroin). And she (the minister's wife) brought my mattress and furniture. And I saw her and she gave me compassion, but at the same time I was still using so it didn't matter, understand, it didn't matter to me. I didn't have the fear of God that I have now. And I did so many, many things that at times I think that God is not going to forgive what I did.]

Music also helped many of the women make it through difficult times. More than one-third of the women (35.8 percent) told us that they used music on a daily basis to help them identify, express, reflect, or relieve their emotions. Their experience and reports to us were consistent with the results of past research. Music stimuli can help individuals understand their own emotional responses by facilitating their experience and identification of emotion; by helping them promote their disclosure of problems, feelings, and thoughts; by facilitating their understanding of others' emotional communications; and by helping them synthesize, control, and modulate their own emotional behavior.[42] Music can actually be therapeutic in that it can help to promote individual growth, insight, and learning; effectuate behavioral change;[43] and, among individuals with severe mental illness, help to reduce psychotic symptoms, improve social functioning, increase individuals' sense of community participation, decrease social isolation, and increase individuals' level of interest in external events.[44]

Maria found encouragement in music to get up and face another day:

"*Me gusta la música a todo volumen.* [I like the music loud.] That makes me feel good, gives me energy." Like many of the women, Maria preferred salsa, merengue, and other Latin music. Salsa, often referred to as the music of barrio people, is a distinct form of music that is closely identified with Puerto Rican culture and is often used as a vehicle for the expression of survival from injustices.[45] This theme resonated with many of the participants who had been in difficult or abusive romantic and sexual relationships. Elena, for instance, explained, "*Me gusta la musica de desprecio.* [I like music about rejection.] I have suffered a lot from rejection and love. I have been betrayed a lot." Hermosa reflected, "I listen to a song called 'Se me rompe el alma' [My Soul Is Breaking] all the time because that is how I feel."

Several of the women used imagery to help them deal with their illness and life's difficulties. Felicita, for instance, imagined that she wore a "Super Mom cape." Although the cape provided her with a positive image, it was not consistently helpful:

> I envision wearing a Super Mom cape. People think I am mental, but I know I am mental anyway. Envisioning this cape works for me, but lately all the stress and fibromyalgia have been affecting me and the cape is not working. I think the cape is broken and it is in the laundry room because I have to sew it or something. . . . I know the difference between a depressive state and when I am past depressed. When I am past depressed, I don't control it, it controls me. It's like stepping out of my body and feeling worthless. Then I am not a good mother; I feel really used.

All of the women who participated in the study had developed some manner of coping, some of which were healthier than others. Their ability to cope with, and in spite of, their mental illness reflects an underlying resilience and offers the potential for further positive growth, which may not even be recognized by the participants themselves. For many of the women, however, this potentiality was restricted and impeded by multiple forces external to them and beyond their control. These circumstances—economic, political, legal, religious, and cultural—and the women's efforts to overcome them are the focus of the chapters that follow.

3

Making Ends Meet

I feel like a *cucaracha en un baile de gallina*
[a roach in a chicken dance].
—Yadra, speaking about her relations with co-workers

Obtaining Employment

Yadra had been able to secure employment despite her diagnoses of major depression, posttraumatic stress disorder, and agoraphobia. She had "beaten the odds," so to speak, unlike the 75 to 85 percent of people in the United States with a severe mental illness who are unable to find work[1] because of their illness symptoms, the side effects of their medication, stigma, discrimination, and employer attitudes toward and expectations of mentally ill people.[2] Yadra's success was all the more remarkable because she was Puerto Rican and, as a minority person with a mental illness, the odds of finding employment were clearly against her.[3]

Migration, Economics, and Racism

Yadra had come to Cleveland from Puerto Rico during a time of "revolving door migration," the most recent of the three periods of migration from Puerto Rico to the U.S. mainland.[4] This period has been so labeled because of the fluctuations in net migration of Puerto Ricans between the U.S. mainland and Puerto Rico and their dispersion into many areas of the mainland outside of the urban areas, such as New York City, where many had originally settled.

The first period of migration, which stretched roughly from 1900 to 1945 and followed the period of the U.S. military occupation of Puerto Rico, has been called the period of the pioneers.[5] Many of these first emigrants likely came from more rural areas of Puerto Rico, where they were small farmers or agricultural laborers on U.S.-owned plantations that had been established for the benefit of their U.S. investors.[6] Significant educational, monetary, legal, and economic modifications had been imposed on Puerto Rico by the United States in order to further even more the investment of U.S. capital and the establishment of North American corporations on the island. These efforts included the devaluation of the local currency and the development of new school curricula to Americanize the population and inculcate U.S. values.[7] As a result of these actions, Puerto Rico's economy was quickly transformed from one in which households grew the food that they consumed to one that was dependent on the United States even for the importation of food that had once been grown there. U.S. bureaucrats attributed the resulting poverty not to the effects of U.S. policies and investments but rather to the island's overpopulation and the idleness of its residents. The only solution, opined the U.S.-appointed governor Arthur Yager in 1915, would be "the transfer of large numbers of Porto [*sic*] Ricans to some other region."[8]

The majority of these emigrants established themselves in various sections of New York City, including the Atlantic Avenue section of Brooklyn, the Lower East Side, Chelsea, the Upper West Side, the Lincoln Center area, and the South Bronx. Many arrived in response to solicitations by corporations for industrial and agricultural labor.[9] It was during this period that Puerto Ricans first migrated to Ohio, growing from a population of 11 in 1910 to 124 by 1920.

The second period, known as "the great migration," spanned from 1946 to 1964. During the fifteen years that immediately followed World War II, an average of forty thousand people left Puerto Rico each year for the U.S. mainland.[10] During this time, the already-settled areas of New York City expanded in size and additional settlements were established in New Jersey, Chicago, and other areas of the country. The Puerto Rican population of Ohio grew to several thousand as increasing numbers of individuals were recruited to the state's steel mills, first from the farms of Michigan and Pennsylvania, where they had originally settled, and then directly from the island.[11] Puerto Rican workers (known as Boricuas) at the National Tube Company in Lorain, Ohio, named their community "La Colonia."

Several theories have been propounded to explain the continuing exodus throughout this period from the island to the mainland. One theory, advanced by Chenault and Handlin, maintains that emigration constituted a solution to excess population that had been brought about by U.S.-formulated improvements in health and medicine.[12] Because the needs of this increased population could not be met, emigration provided an adequate, albeit temporary, solution. Other researchers have argued that the existence of employment opportunities outside of Puerto Rico, many of which were created by mainland U.S. companies seeking temporary workers, "pulled" individuals from Puerto Rico.[13] Still others have maintained that the high rate of emigration was attributable to the inadequacy of the profitable and otherwise successful sugar cane industry in generating sufficient employment, which forced Puerto Rican workers to relocate in order to survive.[14] The Depression, in particular, heralded a contraction of Puerto Rico's agricultural sector, a decline in Puerto Rican incomes, and an increasing dependence on the United States. Structural unemployment increased and many individuals were reduced to part-time work.

Like Yadra, much of Ohio's Puerto Rican population arrived during the third epoch, which roughly spanned the period from 1970 to 2000. During this time, Ohio's Puerto Rican population grew from 21,147 to 66,269. During these same years, Cleveland's Puerto Rican population increased from 8,104 to 25,385, and Lorain's Puerto Rican population almost doubled, growing from 6,031 to 10,536.[15]

Although many minority groups in the United States advanced economically during the 1960s, Puerto Ricans, on the whole, failed to do so.[16] Compared to other Hispanic groups, Puerto Ricans were the only Hispanics who did not narrow the income gap relative to non-Hispanic whites during the 1970s.[17] In fact, the gap widened even further by 1980. Of Puerto Rican families with children, almost half were headed by a woman, and 75 percent of these female-headed households had incomes below the poverty level.[18] By 1987, the median family income for Puerto Ricans was less than half of that for non-Hispanic whites.[19] Employment rates among Puerto Ricans in 1980 were lower than those of any other Hispanic group, and even those who were employed worked fewer hours on average.[20] In 1989, 23.7 percent of all Hispanics living on the U.S. mainland were living below the poverty level. Compared to other Hispanic groups, the proportion of those living below the poverty level was highest among Puerto Ricans (30.8 percent).[21]

Even in more recent years, Puerto Ricans remain relatively poor, both on the island and on the mainland. As of the 1990 census, slightly more than one-third of mainland Puerto Rican individuals lived below the poverty level, while 58.9 percent of individuals on the island lived below the poverty level. As of 1998, 30.9 percent of mainland Puerto Ricans were living in poverty, the highest proportion of any Hispanic/Latino group. Among families, slightly less than one-quarter were living in poverty.[22] This unabated and enduring poverty has been referred to as the "persistent disadvantage" of Puerto Ricans[23] and has been attributed, at least in part, to "official insensitivity, coupled with private and public acts of discrimination."[24]

These conditions are mirrored in the six counties that composed the site of this study. In 1999, the median income for Hispanic-headed households in Cuyahoga County was $29,466, or $15,209 less than the $44,675 median income of white-headed households. In Cleveland, where 41.5 percent of the 478,403 residents are white and 7.3 percent are Hispanic, almost one-third (32.6 percent) of Hispanics live below the poverty level, compared to 16.6 percent of non-Hispanic whites.[25] In Lorain County, where Latinos constitute 6.91 percent of the population, the median household income among Puerto Ricans is $34,231, in comparison with the county-wide median income of $52,856.[26]

Like many of the Puerto Ricans living in northeast Ohio, Yadra had limited education, limited job skills, and limited English ability. As a result, her employment possibilities were severely restricted, even apart from the impact of her mental illness symptoms. Puerto Ricans migrating to Ohio from the island had once been able to find good paying jobs in the state's steel mills. However, the U.S. economic recession of the 1980s brought about a decreased demand for agricultural and industrial labor that resulted in layoffs and increased unemployment rates, both on the mainland and the island. Unemployment and poverty have continued to worsen in recent decades, particularly for Puerto Ricans, as industries have gradually left Ohio's highly populated urban areas to re-establish in lower-wage locales or have vanished altogether, as did the steel mills.[27]

In view of Yadra's own limitations and the limited employment opportunities in the Ohio job market for someone with her skills, it was quite a coup for her to be able to secure employment at a factory. But the atmosphere there was oppressive; she felt the effects of being a Spanish-speaking Puerto Rican woman in a factory dominated by burly, back-slapping white men. She described the misery that she felt on her first day on the job: "I could not stop crying. All of my co-workers laughed at me because the machine pieces I work with are bigger than me. They think it is really funny. I don't let them see my frustration. I laugh back at them so they don't get to me."

Some of her co-workers, she said, were racist. She described one incident when her co-worker committed a "*puerca en el trabajo*" (dirty trick on the job): "A white guy was supposed to teach me how to assemble a piece. He showed me and then I did one and showed him. He told me that I did it well. So I went to continue doing the work and assembled a bunch of pieces. Then the man went and told the supervisor that I had assembled all the pieces wrong. I was cursing the man out in Spanish because he set me up."

Yadra's experience of racism is one that is shared by many individuals of lower socioeconomic status and darker skin color and one that is all too familiar to Puerto Ricans in northeastern Ohio.[28] Puerto Ricans began to experience racism in this region shortly after they first began migrating to the area. Puerto Ricans were initially portrayed during the late 1940s by both the local media and the employers who had recruited them from the island to work in Ohio's steel mills as hardworking, law abiding, and attractive. However, hostility toward the Puerto Rican migrants gradually increased as Ohio's demand for imported labor for its steel mills decreased and the size of the Puerto Rican community grew. No longer welcome, the typical Puerto Rican was then depicted as poorly educated and not particularly conscientious. By the early 1950s, signs appeared on rental housing proclaiming, "NO PUERTO RICANS, NO PETS." A three-faceted program was instituted by both Lorain County and the state of Ohio to discourage further influx of Puerto Ricans into the area, including (1) newspaper announcements indicating that the city of Lorain was unable to accommodate any additional Puerto Rican newcomers; (2) the relocation of Puerto Ricans by Ohio Employment Services to other Ohio cities, including Cleveland and Youngstown; and (3) the institution by social service agencies of workshops designed to discourage Puerto Rican migrants from bringing their family members to the area.[29]

Welfare-to-Work, Not Well Fare

Despite Yadra's efforts to see her illness as only one aspect of who she is, an attitude that appears to be critical for individuals with severe mental illness in obtaining and retaining employment, Yadra ultimately quit her job because of what she called her "nerve condition."[30] In this respect, she is like many women with a severe mental illness. Even when someone with a severe mental illness is able to obtain employment, it may be difficult for them to maintain it because of the fluctuating nature of their illness symptoms, difficulties relating to co-workers, and problems managing both time and stress.[31] The absence of workplace adjustments, such as flexible hours, longer and more frequent breaks, regular supervision and feedback, and sufficient time off for health-related appointments, further decrease the likelihood that someone like Yadra will be able to continue employment.[32] Yadra explained, defeatedly, "*Yo no puedo salir. Me siento inútil. Yo soy joven, puñeta!*" (I can't go out. I feel useless. Fuck, I am young!)

Yadra applied for cash assistance, Medicaid, social security disability, and food stamps, hoping that these benefits would be sufficient to cover the costs of rent, utilities, and food, not only for herself and her three children but also for her sister's three children who were living with her. Yadra's sister, Margarita, who had been diagnosed with a substance use disorder, had begun using heroin again. Workers from child protective services had recommended that Margarita's children be removed from the home permanently after several failed attempts at recovery and her continuing neglect of her children. Even with all of her own financial worries and mental health issues, Yadra had agreed to assume responsibility for her niece and two nephews, believing that it was her obligation as a family member.

Despite Yadra's documented psychiatric history and multiple diagnoses, her application for disability was denied. She became increasingly depressed and found her sessions with her mental health social worker less than helpful: "*David no me entiende. El me desespera. El menos que busco es a David.*" (David does not understand me. He frustrates me. The last person I go to is David.) Part of Yadra's frustration, she explained, was that she needed to express her feelings in Spanish. David could not respond to her until he had looked up the words she used in the Spanish-English/English-Spanish dictionary that he kept on his desk for that purpose. That happened with almost every sentence that she uttered.

Yadra was told to attend a "job club" and an English class as a condition of receiving cash assistance. These requirements were mandated through the welfare-to-work plan that had been established as part of the effort to reform the welfare system.[33] The job club was designed to teach participants how to complete an employment application, compose a resume, conduct themselves during an interview, and dress for work. Yadra's first day at the job club opened with an introduction by the facilitator, recorded directly by the study ethnographer. The facilitator proceeded without pausing for either breath or questions:

> Would everyone please look for your name on the sign-in sheet. In order to get cash assistance, you have to be working at least thirty hours if you are single and thirty-five hours if you are married. The goal of this program is to help you gain the skills needed as far as building your resume. We send you out to volunteer at nonprofit organizations in order to enhance your skills and so you can have experience to note on your resume. We do not place people in places they do not want to be in. We want you to succeed. We try to fit people as best as we can. For some placements such as day cares and schools you will be required to undergo a background check. County background checks only cost six cents and statewide are fifteen cents. Remember that when we place you somewhere it does not mean that place is going to hire you. I am a true testament of this program. I was in this program five years ago, and I was lucky enough to get hired. It is not set in stone that the organizations are going to hire you, but if you do a good job they might just want to keep you. You will be receiving a referral letter with the contact person that you need to reach at the site. It will also have your start date. You need to show up on time every day. If you cannot show up for a just reason, you need to call the contact person. Make sure that you have good grooming habits when you go to the site. For women we have a program called Dress for Success that helps you learn what to wear, and the program for men is called Career Gear. Make sure you come with a positive attitude.
>
> When I mentioned earlier that in order to miss you must have just cause, this is what I mean: You have medical documentation to give the site. Keep a copy for yourself. Another just cause would be a death. You can only be out for a maximum of five days. You must also provide a letter from the funeral home. If you are incarcerated you will need to be reinstated when you get out. And the last reason is if you are going to employment interviews.
>
> On to transportation and day care. You will be receiving an additional fifty-four dollars on your check. This money is for a bus pass if you need one. For day care you will be getting a day care voucher.

> You will also get a listing of providers that will be given to you by your worker. The day care vouchers will also come from your worker.
>
> Not complying with these rules will result in you being sanctioned. . . . For your first sanction it will be a month without a check. You must go ten days to your WEP [Work Experience Program] assignment and cannot miss not one day during sanction. For the second offense you will be sanctioned three months with no check or food stamps. Then for the third offense you will be sanctioned six months. Your check, food stamps, and medical will be taken away.
>
> As soon as you become employed you must notify your worker and your supervisor at your WEP site. We recommend that you do not jump into a job that you are really not going to like. Make it a sound decision so you will be successful because if you quit employment without just cause that can also get you into trouble. You will not be able to receive services for six months other than medical for the kids. Just cause for leaving employment would have to be one of the following: employment is unsuitable due to pay decreases, wages are under federal minimum, the work site is subject to a health strike, unsafe work environment, and lack of supportive services.
>
> Tomorrow there is an optional career center orientation at nine o'clock. You are more than welcome to come to that. They will be testing for math and reading skill levels.
>
> We have concluded the first part of the orientation. Now I will have a one-on-one interview with each of you in which we will discuss placement. Remember that you have access to this room Monday through Friday from seven to four. You have access to the computers and can use the phones to make calls related to employment. Internet is also available for job search and work-related reasons. Someone is always available at this lab to help with questions. No food or drinks are permitted in here. During our one-on-one interview I will once again go over your rights and responsibilities.

Yadra told her case worker that she wanted to go to work on an assembly line but was informed that that kind of work didn't meet the requirements of the assistance program. She was also told that she would have to work thirty-five hours a week, notwithstanding her mental illness and her many appointments with her psychiatrist, her mental health social worker, and her gynecologist, who had recently discovered what appeared to be the early signs of uterine cancer. When Yadra was sanctioned by her case worker for missing a "work and training orientation" session, she felt like her world was closing in on her: "I don't know what is wrong with me. I have been crying [for days]. I got a sanction letter from the social worker. . . . I wanted to kill myself. And it's not the kids that make me feel this way. It is the adults that give me problems and grief. I was so stressed out. . . . I have even been thinking of calling [my psychiatrist] and asking him to lock me up for at least three days."

The team ethnographer Juanita brought Yadra to the psychiatric unit of a major hospital, where she was evaluated by another social worker for suicide risk. In response to the questions posed by the hospital social worker, Yadra explained, "My plan was to cut my jugular. *Porque quiero morir. Porque no valgo na.* [Because I want to die. Because I am not worth anything.] The only thing with any worth is my children." Yadra remained in the hospital for four days, longer than the seventy-two-hour hold that was required by law for observation of individuals who are believed to be at risk of committing suicide or harming others. When she was released, she felt better, but her relief was momentary, lasting only until she became aware of the morass of bureaucratic paperwork and battles that lay before her. Her welfare worker had closed her case and terminated her food stamps and cash assistance. After all, Yadra had once again failed to appear at the job club. Yadra's claim for disability had also been denied again. Distraught, she cried,

> *Todo me sale mal. Mi vida no tiene sentido. Yo no me quiero matar. Es que no puedo estar sola. Ahí es cuando me viene esa cosa que yo no puedo controlar. Pues como cortarme las venas, a que hora, como, cuando no haiga nadie en la casa. Si los nenes no estuvieran, mi vida es mierda. Tengo miedo que no este en suerte y que no puede parar los pensamientos.* [Everything comes out wrong. My life has no purpose. I don't want to kill myself. I just can't be alone. That is when that thing comes over me. Well, like cutting my wrist, at what time, like, when no one is at the house. If the children were not around, my life is shit. I am scared that I will run out of luck and not be able to stop the thoughts.]

Retaining Employment

Like Yadra, Catalina had migrated to Cleveland from Puerto Rico. Also like Yadra, she spoke primarily Spanish and had only a high school education. Catalina also suffered from major depression, as did Yadra, but her symptoms were not as severe and she had developed positive strategies to manage the ups and downs of everyday life. Catalina was grateful that she had been able to find a housekeeping job with a major medical institution, but was concerned about her ability to retain her employment because of her physical health:

> I don't know what I am going to do about work, too, because the doctor has given me some restrictions. The job does not accept those restrictions. I cannot lift anything over thirty pounds. If I am on my feet I need to take frequent breaks. *Yo lo cojo suave.* [I take it easy.] I sit when I am tired. If the supervisor passes by I tell them my legs hurt. The other day I had really bad pain in my legs. I went to the atrium at work and lay down on a sofa. The supervisor just then passed by and saw me. I told him I was in pain. He was not too happy with me.

Her job became more difficult emotionally after she was unexpectedly confronted with the death of her nephew:

> Emotionally I do not feel good. . . . I don't know for how long I can stay working there because of my health condition. . . . I do not like having to go to the morgue. That smell makes me sick. Then they don't really explain to you what you need to do in the area so you have to figure it out by yourself. In the morgue there is a long table. In the sink there is a hose that sucks out the blood from the dead bodies. You see jars of brains and body organs. Then there are buckets everywhere of the stuff they take out. It is disgusting. One day I was working in the emergency room and my nephew came in through the trauma unit. He was having convulsions and died. He was only two and a half years old. I don't like working there because it reminds me of his death.

Catalina had many family stresses to deal with in addition to her own challenges managing her mental illness, her physical health, and the demands of her job. Her twenty-six-year-old son, whom she had had at a young age, was in prison in Puerto Rico. His ten-year sentence for cocaine use had been reduced to five years, but Catalina said he was in a bad way. Her younger son Nestor, one of three children living with her, also suffered from depression. He had become aggressive, Catalina said, and constantly got into fights at school. At one point, he was removed from her home and placed in an institution for delinquent minors. He was back home now, but it seemed that he had turned his anger inward on himself, instead of lashing out at others as before. Catalina was at her wit's end:

> I can't go on like this with this kid. Yesterday he tried to hang himself. I had to take the rope from his neck. [The doctors] gave him some pills. The pills take away his appetite. They say he is going through a major depression. . . . I do not know what I am going to do with him. We had a meeting at the school to see if they can help him. They are going to place him in special education classes. The lawyer from SSI [social security income] attended the meeting and said he thinks that Nestor will be eligible for SSI benefits.

The SSI benefits would help Catalina out a lot, she observed. Even though she received several hundred dollars a month in food stamps, her paychecks from work were still not enough to pay for the other expenses for herself and her kids. She was divorced from her husband, the father of the three children who lived with her, and he had long been absent from her life emotionally, physically, and financially. She was already planning to move to a smaller apartment, where the rent would be only $400 a month. It would be the fifth move for the family in less than three years, and she was not happy that they would have to move yet again. She also had lots of bills to worry about. Nestor needed a root canal, which was going to cost her $370 that she did not have. Even though she had health insurance for herself and her children through her work, the insurance company had not paid the hospital bill for her daughter, and the hospital was billing her for $770; she had decided to cancel her daughter's follow-up appointment because she couldn't face another bill. Catalina's driver's license had been suspended, but she couldn't get it reinstated until she was able to save enough to pay all of the fines that she owed.

Catalina talked periodically about possibly quitting her job because of her health and the additional stress that it caused her. It's possible, though, that her employment actually helped her to deal with the many and varied demands on her time and attention. In addition to providing her with a stable income, it is likely that her success in the competitive world of work boosted her self-esteem so that she could address these other issues, feeling competent rather than overwhelmed.[34] Catalina's participation in the world of work allowed her the opportunity to establish relationships with individuals outside of her usual sphere of reference, to play a role in the economic system, and to assume the status possessed by those with purchasing power.[35] Unemployment could result in a contraction of her social network and a diminishment of her self-esteem, leading to further deterioration of her mental health.[36]

Although benefits like SSI, food stamps, and cash assistance helped some of the women to make ends meet, the requirements imposed by some of the programs seemed to some of the women to be short-sighted, demeaning, and inhumane. Yadra's benefits, for instance, had been cut off when she missed a training session because she had been hospitalized for her depression and threat of suicide. Cesara's feelings about "the system" were similar to Yadra's. Cesara was receiving food stamps and cash assistance for herself and her three children and had been told that she had to find a job. Her job prospects were limited given her high school education, her relative lack of English, and the recurring symptoms of her bipolar disorder. She saw no point in obtaining a minimum wage job in a service industry, which she would be likely to lose in only a short time because of Cleveland's worsening economy. She wanted, instead, to be able to receive training that would provide her with a more solid foundation in life. Her welfare worker had even threatened to have her benefits cut off because she had failed to attend several job orientation classes, even though she had been at the doctor's office on those days and had provided written notes from her physician verifying that that was where she was. The system, she thought, was racist and stacked against her:

> I want to go to school but they sent me to [a] job search. I asked if I can go to nursing school training. They said no. They don't care about Hispanics. They only help blacks and whites. They kill my strength to go to school. They don't support you in anything. *A mi me da lo mismo.* [I don't care.] I don't care. I could not go to work when I was pregnant. I wanted to go to school and they didn't allow it. They sent me to vocational guidance. They think since I have three kids I'm the one in need. If I was black they will help. They are racist toward Latinos. I'll be OK. I'll be at a shelter with food for my kids. Everyone is pressuring me. They don't know how I feel. I went to [my social worker]. He said I put too many excuses. I don't have a car. Now I know why people are alcoholics and prostitutes. They say I'm young but I have three kids. Family doesn't help. I get tired sometimes. My family make fun of me.

> Sometimes I want to be gone for twenty-four hours. Just hang out, see if I find myself. They think I'm lazy. They don't know how I feel. They judge me.

Even with all of the hours shadowing Cesara, it was hard to know sometimes whether her perceptions were colored by her sometimes-occurring paranoia and delusions. However, at least one study of welfare reform and the job club suggests that Spanish-speaking women have often been denied vocational training and are steered instead into part-time, low-wage, or temporary positions.[37] Nevertheless, Cesara had discovered ways to make the system work for her. Food stamps, she found, could be used to serve multiple functions: "Yes, I buy a lot of food [with food stamps], sell some to my brother. I hate to sell food stamps but sometimes I have to do it so I can pay a bill. The kids don't eat a lot, and I get plenty of milk from the WIC [Women, Infants, and Children program]. My refrigerator doesn't work too well so I gave my sister the WIC coupons. I also get money from welfare for transportation."[38]

Scraping By

Honoria was not able to work at all. She had once worked at two jobs, cleaning hotel rooms. At that time, she said, she was always busy. She had never finished high school, but her English was good and she was a hard worker. In those days, she weighed 160 pounds, but now, on her medication for her mental illness, she had put on so much weight that she said of herself, "I'm so fat I look like that thing in Star Wars. Jabba the Hutt." She said of her life before her diagnosis of bipolar disorder, "I used to go out and drink Coronas, mixed drinks, and tequila with my friends. It was fun. . . . I was bad. I drank and smoked. . . . I used men. I never felt real feelings for men, only my husband. I like the way I dressed and the energy I had. I can't explain it to you." Honoria had used drugs extensively back in those days, but had given it up.

Honoria relied on social security. It was enough, she said, to pay her bills and buy her food. This was possible only because Honoria was so frugal and careful with money; a large proportion of individuals subsisting on social security are unable to make it through an entire month after paying for their rent and food.[39] She lived with her husband, Alfredo, but he used a separate address for official purposes. They had previously used the same address, but the amount of public assistance they each received had been reduced because they were living in the same household. Honoria had then told her husband to find a different address so that she could get her full benefits. She wasn't quite sure what he did with all of his money. She knew that he used part of it to buy alcohol and weed. He was back on heroin as well, which scared her:

> He is sick [points to her arm]. He needs some. When I got pregnant he was clean, but now he is back on it so I haven't slept with him. I get scared, sleeping with him, because that is a chemical he puts in the body. His blood needs it, he gets diarrhea and everything. He was clean and now he is back on it. Pretty soon he'll leave and invent something. I thought he would change because I'm pregnant, but he hasn't changed.

Honoria stopped taking her antidepressants when she found out that she was pregnant. She was concerned about the effect that they might have on her soon-to-be-born child.[40] She hadn't told her doctor that she had stopped using them, though. Instead, she gave them to her husband to sell on the street. He could get two dollars for every pill, so it was extra money in his pocket. Honoria never saw any of the money.

Many of the other women in the study were unable to find and maintain legal employment of any kind, for many of the same reasons: limited education and job skills, a lack of previous employment history, and symptoms of their mental illness. It is also possible that some of the women were discouraged from seeking employment because they believed that they would not find work or that they could not work because of their mental illness. This self-devaluation can be a secondary effect of being labeled with a mental illness diagnosis and the stereotypes associated with that diagnosis.[41] This occurs through a process by which

> individuals who become mental patients may devalue themselves because they now belong to a category that they believe most people view negatively. . . . Patients may be concerned about how others will respond to them and therefore engage in defenses that lead to strained interaction, isolation, and other negative consequences. In the first case, self-concept and self-esteem are affected as people turn the perceived negative views of others onto themselves. In the second, the process of "imaginative rehearsal" causes individuals to be constrained by their

> perceptions of others' likely responses to them. These two processes are closely intertwined.[42]

This process could affect a woman's search for work in several ways. First, she might self-isolate or associate only with those individuals who are also mentally ill, thereby limiting the possibility of finding gainful and meaningful employment. Alternatively, she might proactively try to educate a new employer about the illness, but even if successful, this strategy could result in a loss of leverage, rather than enhanced understanding and flexibility. In fact, neither strategy has been found to work very well.[43] In such circumstances, having a mental illness may ultimately be an "engulfing role" or "master status," becoming the focus of the individual's identity and existence.[44]

For many of the women, the conflation of these barriers increasingly appeared to be insurmountable as Cleveland's economy worsened and the labor market became more competitive and dominated by service industries that demanded personal interaction between their employees and their clientele.[45] For some, there were also financial disincentives to work because any job that they might find would pay less than the amount they received each month in benefits. Any value that could be derived from holding a job would hardly offset the lost income and the increased stress that they might feel, having to juggle doctors' appointments, illness symptoms, medication side effects, and the structure of a regular workday.[46]

When drugs were part of the picture, finding work and making ends meet were even more difficult.[47] Only 15 to 35 percent of opiate-addicted individuals are able to find employment, and among severely mentally ill individuals, substance use is one of the major reasons for employment termination.[48] Yadra and Catalina didn't use either alcohol or drugs, and Honoria had given up on both years before. Even though Hermosa had tried several times to kick heroin, she had been unable to stay clean for very long. She was on a waiting list for admission into a residential treatment facility for Latino heroin users, but the wait was so long that, as she put it, she "*mejor yo rompo el vicio en casa*" (might as well break the habit at home). She was trying to cut back on her heroin use and had started buying ten-dollar bags instead of twenty-dollar bags. In addition to the SSI payments that she received because of her bipolar disorder, Hermosa made ends meet by stealing: "*Yo le robaba a mi familia, yo le robaba a mi tía, yo le robaba a cualquiera cuando estaba en eso porque lo necesitaba.*" (I robbed my family, I robbed my aunt, I robbed whoever whenever because I needed it.) She also developed a strategy for obtaining refunds for stolen merchandise as another means of augmenting her income: "*Miro, yo iba a* [name of store] *y robaba la mercancía. . . .* Easy, *yo buscaba el dinero. Sin el recibo. Con mi* ID." (Look, I went to the store, I stole, and I looked for the money. Easy, I looked for a refund. Without a receipt. With my ID.) If research is to be believed, rather than stereotypical images and popular belief, it is unlikely that Hermosa's receipt of SSI contributed to the amount of her drug use.[49]

Delfina had developed similar strategies. She prided herself on having stolen items valued at more than $10,000 from stores while she was pregnant, hiding them in her "belly." Although she was currently working at a topless bar, earning about $250 a night, she worked only when she needed the money: "I only dance when I want to and when I need the money. I've been dancing since I was eighteen years old. I've been dancing every day, seven days a week, and I used to dance in New York and make good money. I don't like dancing without my clothes." She explained that she often used glitter to cover her breasts and nipples so that she would not feel naked. Delfina, who was raised in the Pentecostal faith, wanted to stop dancing and go back to church. Even so, the dancing was an easy way to raise extra cash, and she found it difficult to leave the excitement of that life. Delfina had been diagnosed with bipolar disorder; it seemed that her manic phases provided her with the frenetic energy that she needed to dance for the nine long hours of her shift, until 2:30 in the morning. Delfina was contemptuous of women who relied on men for their support: "Man, summertime is coming and Cleveland is dirty, women looking for pockets. . . . They walk around like hoochies now. I don't want a man. I think I'll be by myself, feels better. These women throw themselves at my man. They don't care." Even so, Delfina, like Hermosa, was willing to trade sex with men in exchange for gifts and money to pay her bills, her alcohol, and her street drugs.

The scene was completely different during her depressed periods, though, when getting out of bed felt as if she were rising from the dead. During these episodes, Delfina had so little energy that she was unable to do much of anything. She left raw meat to rot on the table, and her three children's spits of toothpaste remained as decorations on her walls for weeks at a time.

Several women would have earned Delfina's contempt if they had known each other. Jimena depended on her mother's boyfriend Oscar's check to pay the bills and his Section 8 housing to put a roof over their heads.[50] She frequented the church next door for bags of food. Katia, too, often relied on men to fill in the gaps in her income. She had once worked in clubs as a stripper, earning up to $600 in one night. She was looking for work now as a clerical assistant. In the interim, until she found a decent paying job, she relied on social security benefits that she received because the symptoms of her bipolar disorder often interfered with her ability to remain employed on those relatively few occasions when she had been able to find a job. Katia supplemented that income through other activities. She had periodically worked for a small shop owner, cleaning machines and cooking for him. He had often rewarded her with small bonuses, like five dollars so that she could buy cigarettes for herself. She lost that job, though, after he was robbed and held her responsible for it.

Katia still enjoyed going out to clubs, but her income from benefits wouldn't stretch far enough to pay for her drinks or a cover charge. Katia laughed as she explained how she was able to get a man to cover her drinks:

> You need to walk up to the men and just talk to them. You can't look like you got money. You need to act like a bitch and tease them, talk nasty to them. *Yo le monto el labio.* [I put my lip on him.] Guys buy me drinks but if they think you have money, they won't buy you anything. I always tell them I am thirsty [*laughing*]. If you ever need money, hook up with a married man because they'll give you money and they won't bother you.

Katia was similarly able to obtain an apartment without paying rent, through the male friend of a male friend. Katia also frequented the streets of Lakewood, a small city immediately west of downtown Cleveland, on Wednesday nights because that was when residents put out their garbage for pickup the following morning. She often found barely worn and highly desirable shoes, shirts, and curtains that had been laid out on the curbs. She found ways to make her money go furthest, as when she purchased a car radio for only $25: "This brand of radio is the best. I got it from drug people, they want fast money."

Some of the women, like Sabrina, a middle-aged woman with a longstanding history of bipolar disorder, resorted to sex work in an effort to make ends meet. Sabrina explained to Isa why she and her then-current boyfriend had begun sex work:

> At times he would do sexual favors for men in order to get his fix [drugs]. I told him I understood that because at times, I too exchanged sexual favors for drugs. *Aunque no me pare en la esquina. Yo llamaba desde mi casa pero soy igual y es lo mismo de la que se para en la esquina.* [Even though I did not stand at a corner. I would call from my house, I am the same and it is the same thing as the one that stands on the corner.]

Sabrina knew enough about HIV to ask her boyfriend if the sores on his skin might be a sign of the infection. He assured her that it was a bad case of psoriasis. That scare, however, did not convince her to use condoms with her sex clients, perhaps because the money was better without condoms.

True, it was Sabrina's decision not to use a condom, to leave herself vulnerable to the possibility of contracting HIV. She was complicit in this dynamic of care and collusion with her boyfriend, a dynamic characterized by mutual affection and warmth, but one that often centered on the need to maintain their addictions.[51] Although Sabrina's choices were hers, they were nevertheless constrained by the intersecting and simultaneously occurring forces that remained well beyond her control and yet affected her everyday existence—regional poverty, high unemployment, gender inequity, racism, lack of adequate recovery services—all manifestations of structural violence.[52] (Structural violence is discussed more fully in Chapter 9.)

not left her "so alone" and had paid more attention to her, then she hung up on him. Her husband called her back from Puerto Rico, begging for her forgiveness, saying that he had not known she was feeling this way, and promising to be home within a matter of hours.

The drama did not end there. Javier Cristobal moved in with Isabella, her husband, and their three children. Then Isabella discovered that Javier Cristobal was in the United States illegally, and decided to divorce her husband and marry Javier Cristobal so that he could obtain legal status through her. Isabella represented the situation to her husband as simply a temporary arrangement to help out a friend who had decided to relocate, an accommodation for friends and family members that is quite common. Nevertheless, her husband may have sensed that Isabella was more involved emotionally with Javier Cristobal than she was acknowledging, telling her that she was "crazy with this whole situation." Isabella confided to one of the ethnographers:

JUANITA: So, Isabella, let me ask you a question. Are you still planning to move forward with the divorce to help Javier Cristobal?

ISABELLA: Yes, we still have those plans. I need help filling out the papers of the dissolution of marriage.

JUANITA: How do you feel about all of this?

ISABELLA: *No te puedo negar que estoy enamorada de el.* [I cannot deny that I am in love with him.]

JUANITA: Is your husband aware of your feelings towards Javier Cristobal?

ISABELLA: He has no need to know that. No one needs to know that. I really don't know what is going to happen with all of this.

JUANITA: So what is the purpose of getting the dissolution of marriage?

ISABELLA: The purpose still is to help Javier Cristobal get his papers to stay in this country. The rest we will just have to wait and see.

It was never completely clear what Isabella meant when she said they would "have to wait and see." Nevertheless, from our vantage point, based on the information that Isabella had been willing to divulge, it looked very much as if she had set her sights on a new life with Javier Cristobal, despite the seventeen-year difference in their ages, the illegality of her scheme, and the potential emotional and legal consequences to all concerned. Her husband was not opposed to the divorce, although we could not know whether his apparent resignation to the situation was due to his frustration with Isabella and her ever-present depression, his dismay at her involvement with another man, or the guilty belief, inculcated and constantly reinforced by Isabella, that his inattentiveness to her needs was responsible for her abandonment of their marriage.

Ultimately, the couple did not divorce, Javier Cristobal left Cleveland for parts unknown, and Isabella abandoned her fantasy of moving herself and her children to South Carolina or Virginia to be with him. Isabella and her husband settled back into their once-familiar routines of daily living. Isabella's husband continued to provide her with the financial and emotional stability and safety that she so desperately needed, yet had been willing to forsake in exchange for some momentary excitement and an escape from the drudgery of her existence. While Isabella's husband may not have been the perfect mate, and their relationship may not have been ideal, her husband was accepting of her periodic harangues, her emotional infidelity, and her illness and its associated mood swings.

Tainted Love

Many of the women were on one or more occasions involved in relationships that, while not abusive, were clearly not healthy. Many had multiple sexual partners, often without any real emotional involvement. This pattern of multiple sexual partners is often seen among women with histories of incest.[3] A large proportion of the women in this study reported having been sexually abused as children by fathers, brothers, uncles, and/or family "friends," and although many of them also reported having multiple sexual partners, the sexual abuse did not directly cause them to have multiple sexual partners.[4] Their involvement with multiple sexual partners, frequently without the use of condoms, significantly increased their risk of HIV infection and other sexually transmitted infections. (The women's HIV risk is discussed in detail in Chapter 7.)

Maria had been abused sexually by her father and often had flashbacks of the incidents, which she described to us in detail and which had been recorded in her case files throughout the intervening years by the succession of social workers and psychiatrists who had provided her with mental health care. Her first sexual experience with a girl occurred when she was eleven years old. At that young age, she was also having sex with four married men. At the time of our study, she considered herself a very sexual person and was frustrated by her husband's impotence. Her feelings about her sexual experiences were interwoven with the religion-oriented hallucinations of her schizophrenia:

> I've slept with a lot of people and don't want to cheat on my husband. I never used anything [condom] with the men I slept with. The other night I had a dream I was having sex with a plastic demon. In the name of God I am going to get the sexual demons out of my house. I can smell them and see them when they are inside my house. People sometimes bring sexual spirits [demons] with them in my home; I can see them in people. I am very careful who I bring in my house. I eventually get them all out of the house *con ayuno y oracion* [with prayer and fasting]. God always takes care of me at all times and protected me from getting AIDS. Back then I slept with men because I didn't know sex was a bad thing. We [she and her husband] use each other's hand for pleasure. The women I slept with were friends. I wonder how it would be to be with a woman now. Women understand better than men. . . . A lot of black angels are walking around. The black angels are lost souls in the streets. They walk the streets looking for forgiveness because they want to live. Reincarnation, that's the reason why we have to also pray for the dead. A lot of people go to see psychics, and God doesn't like that. The souls are people who are dead, who enter animals' bodies like a body of a cat to walk the streets. Everyone wants to be saved and sometimes they are stuck in the streets so the demons possess them. If we pray for the dead, God will hear us. Kids who die and are under nine years old go straight to heaven because they haven't sinned yet. The dark angels also use people's bodies, they enter people's bodies who have mental illnesses, people who are in psychiatric facilities, and homeless people. They also enter bodies of emotionally abused and sexual offenders. *Las almas estan torturadas.* [The souls are being tortured.] I don't judge people, but prostitutes have a evil spirit of sexuality, it's a bad spirit. I struggle with this spirit.[5]

Maria talked frequently about the orgies that she attended. Like several of the other women, she was aware of the HIV risk associated with having had unprotected sexual relations with multiple partners, but refused to be tested. Maria was especially worried that she may have had sex with an HIV-positive person and believed that she would likely become infected if she was not already. Maria's brother, who became HIV-infected through injection drug use, died of AIDS.

Natalia was raped by her father when she was eighteen. Since that time, she had heard his voice speaking to her. She was also beaten by both parents. She had used crack, cocaine, marijuana, and alcohol in the past, and continued to use alcohol and marijuana. She had frequent hallucinations and had made many suicide attempts that necessitated hospitalization. Natalia had never been married but had had numerous male and female sexual partners. She had been arrested on at least one occasion for harassment and had difficulty controlling her own violent behavior. She was very worried that she would become infected with HIV if she was not already, and believed that she had probably had sexual relations with someone who was HIV-positive. She refused to be tested, however, because she did not believe that the results were really kept confidential or anonymous. Like many other unemployed Puerto Rican women with relatively little education, Natalia did not want to use condoms during sex.[6] She believed that using a condom meant she could not trust her partner. She never asked partners, male or female, whether they had been tested for HIV.

Laura, who had been diagnosed with bipolar disorder, had had similar abusive experiences. She was sexually abused by several of her family members and, later, was physically abused by her romantic partner. Her experiences had left her distrustful of men in general: "[No] husband or a man [can] tell me what to do. Men come in, stay with you for a long time, use you, rape your daughters, beat you, or cheat on you. The first years are fine and then they start mistreating you. I don't go for that; then they take, you see their claws. They start showing you their nails."

The women's efforts to leave unhealthy relationships were sometimes thwarted by their past lovers. Imelda, who had been diagnosed with schizophrenia, enrolled in the study shortly after she turned eighteen. She had been sexually abused by her grandfather as a child. Imelda had once been a straight-A student, but her grades plummeted after the abuse began and she attempted suicide. She later became involved with a man who she said was obsessed with her and became even more obsessed after she terminated their relationship and became involved with another man. She finally threatened him with a restraining order if he did not leave her alone, explaining to our ethnographer Isa that she had no other choice because "he is a psycho." Like Laura, Imelda had developed a very definite point of view about relationships as a result of her experiences with men:

> Girls in this generation are not going to make it. They are not going to make it to the top because they are in love too young. They don't have a career. They are taking girls. Men are taking girls, all the girls sixteen and over. It's wrong. They should get a vote to have all the girls operated until they are 18. They should not be pregnant so they can go to school and have all the sex they want. They should not fuck up their lives. . . . All the girls should get condoms. I tell every girl that comes here, listen to this, understand this from my mouth. I don't have a job, I don't have a career, I never have any jewelry. I have nothing. You want to be like me, no money, no nothing? Don't have sex. Use condoms. I thank God I never had anything. I took care of myself and I use contraceptives.

Although Imelda asserted that she always used contraceptives and protected herself with condoms, her situation and her actions cast doubt on this representation. Imelda had had three children and periodically went to a publicly funded clinic for HIV and syphilis testing, concerned that she may have contracted either infection from one of her many boyfriends, a near impossibility if she had actually been using condoms during intercourse.

Long Hard Road out of Hell

Many of the women encountered emotional or physical brutality or both in their search for Mr. or Mrs. Right, rather than the love, affection, and companionship that they sought. Yadra explained how she was devastated by yet another criticism from her partner and how it exacerbated the ruminations that were so common to her depression:

> He knows that I suffer from depression and take medications but he does not completely know about my condition and my past. I also do not want to tell him because I don't want him to think that he is superior to me. *El es mujeriego.* [He is a womanizer.] I can tell by his eyes. And the other day he made a comment that upset me a lot. *Me dijo que estaba un poco gordita.* [He told me that I was a bit chubby.] That was worse to me than if he would have insulted me. That is the worst

> thing he could have said. *Yo lo se pero que no me lo diga. Por eso tengo el celebro así. Le doy mucha vuelta a las palabras.* [I know it but he does not have to tell me. That is why my brain is this way. I go around words a lot.]

More than two-thirds of the women in the study (68 percent) had suffered physical partner violence at some point during their lives, and almost one-third (32 percent) were victimized by a partner during the course of the study. The violence ranged in severity from punches and slaps to severe beating and vaginal and anal rape. Unfortunately, such violence is an all-too-common experience for many women with severe mental illness, who may be more vulnerable to partner violence than other women.[7] Although the reasons for this apparent increased vulnerability are unclear, it is thought to be associated with the symptoms and consequences of the mental illness itself, such as impaired judgment, difficulties with planning, difficulties with interpersonal relationships, long-term isolation, and repeated stigmatizing experiences.[8] Cumulatively, these circumstances may foster a willingness to engage in any relationship that offers the possibility of love and acceptance, regardless of the cost.

The violence the women faced sometimes also increased their risk of contracting HIV. This was certainly true of Osana. Osana had been born in Puerto Rico into a Catholic family but had long ago left that faith community. At the time that we first met her, Osana was thirty-seven years old. She could speak some English but frequently alternated between English and Spanish, particularly when she was upset or confused. She had been married to a man in Puerto Rico but had left him to be with Jesus, who had promised her love and loyalty and for whom she had felt a strong sexual attraction. Instead of romance and encouragement, however, she encountered control and confusion. Osana explained what her life with her lover Jesus had been like when they lived together:

> He would always tell me to cover my body up because the man next door was looking at me through the window. The house next door did not have any windows on one side so the man could not possibly look into my bedroom. I felt like a little girl. . . . I could not do anything. One day we were walking down the street when he punched me on my jaw. He accused me of looking at a man sitting on his porch. At first I did not know what hit or why. I felt dizzy and he started yelling at me and calling me a bitch. I could not wake up before him because he

> would beat me. I had to lay there and look at the ceiling. That is the worse feeling in the world. . . . You stare at the walls and ceiling and think about your life a lot. My eyes would not close back up because I was not sleeping, my body was jumpy from lying on the bed. He would put his arm around me to make sure I would not go anywhere.

It was not until Jesus almost killed her that she found the wherewithal to escape. She described the event that finally pushed their relationship over the edge:

> He was asking me for money for drugs. I didn't want to give it to him. . . . On that day he told me to withdraw all the money [from the bank], and I told him I was not going to withdraw the money. He asks for the PIN number and I told him I was not going to give it to him. He started to hit me in the bedroom. After he beats me he starts to cry on top of me and tells me he loves me. After that he tells me to get up and tells me to go with him . . . so I can sell my body. He said, "Since you don't want to give me the money then you need to find it for me because I want to be cured."[9] . . . He tells me to get dressed and he cuts my leg with a knife. . . .
>
> He said if I didn't give him the money I was going to have to sell myself. Well, he takes me and on the way there he beats me. . . . He took me to a bridge where there was a lady doing drugs. . . . I saw she had AIDS, because of her skin condition. He needed a hit [i.e., injection of drugs]! . . . I didn't want to give him the money because . . . I wanted that money to leave him, and then he takes me under the bridge. There was needles, cookers, and capsules, and pills everywhere on the ground. . . . Well this lady was sitting getting a hit. She took out the needle and took out blood. . . . Then she injects herself. She had a small bottle of water and the needle. She told Jesus not to use it and he became aggressive and took it from her, without cleaning it [the needle] or putting it in bleach . . . because they get a kit with bleach with everything. He burned the drug, put water, and he injected it. When I saw that I became hysterical because I said to myself this is crazy . . . because he didn't clean it and that needle automatically would give him hepatitis. He automatically would get hepatitis. For sure he got it. I knew afterwards. I got hysterical and wanted to leave but he didn't let me leave. Well, he started hitting me . . . and the girl would tell him, look she is a nice girl, don't hit her.

> Then she asked me what was I doing with a man like that but I could not say anything. . . .
>
> He starts to look sleepy. I started running but since I'm fat I could not run fast so he caught on to me. When he caught me he started hitting me again. . . . He hit me hard. He got so mad and said, look what I'm going to do to you. He started in this hand with the needle . . . yes, in my face. On the floor. I did not let him, I tried with him but he hit me. He stabbed me with the needle on my hands and thighs. When I felt him stabbing me I thought about the lady he shared the needle with. I thought of her and how I would get AIDS. He already used the needle, had blood contact with this third person and now it's in my blood. I'm sick. I'm fucked up now and going to die. I lost my mind and I told God I did not deserve this. Everything went through my mind. Blood came out but not a large amount because it was a needle not a knife. Then he had cut me with a knife. I was cut up. I said to myself he did that right after taking the needle out of his veins. . . . I was struggling so he would stop. I threw dirt in his eyes, I tried to defend myself. I fell on the floor and there was glass on the floor. I started to cut myself. Because I said to myself I'm already sick. I had no hope. I gave my life to him . . . a lot of things went through my mind. It was like I was going to die.

Osana was able to run from Jesus to a courthouse, where the guard saw that she was injured and being pursued and had Jesus arrested. Even now, years after leaving Jesus, Osana continues to have flashbacks and worries that Jesus will find her when he is released from jail.

In many ways, Osana's horrific experience mirrors that of many abused women in similar circumstances who are not mentally ill. Lower socioeconomic status has been found to be predictive of partner violence, perhaps because of the stress and instability associated with limited financial resources.[10] Alcohol and drug use have also been linked with victimization, both as a stimulus to the perpetration of violence and as a consequence of having been abused.[11] In many cities, including Cleveland, ubiquitous violence and substance abuse, together with the associated HIV risk, are not merely concurrent problems but represent, instead, "a set of mutually reinforcing interconnected epidemics," or a "syndemic."[12] Osana's mental illness symptoms likely limited her opportunities to develop an intimate relationship, while the stigma associated with her mental illness may have narrowed the pool of potential partners.[13]

Lalia was repeatedly raped throughout her relationship with her husband. She was willing to talk about the trauma that she experienced, but would not permit the ethnographer to tape-record the conversation. According to the ethnographer's notes,

> She went to a sexologist where they showed her movies and magazines of a sexual nature and explained to her what her duties were as a wife. She said that her lack of desire in sex made her husband be abusive towards her. She said that when he would get in, he would tear her robe and rape her. She said that he would not stop until she bled. She described an incident that happened when she was nine months pregnant with her first child. He would take her to the room and turn the air conditioner on high. She said the room had Italian tiles on the floor, so he would take her clothes off, rape her and then throw her on the cold floor, naked until the next day.

Lalia's experience is not unique to her alone. Rape and physical abuse of pregnant women by their intimate partners is all too common.[14] In some studies, up to one-third of pregnant women interviewed have reported being sexually abused, and physically abusive partners may escalate their violence in response to the pregnancy.[15] And, although marital rape would likely be traumatic for anyone experiencing it, it may have been particularly devastating for Lalia, who often lacked a cohesive awareness of her surroundings and situation because of the severity of her schizophrenia.

Almost a quarter of the women (22.6 percent) had at some time tried to fight back against a violent partner. Catalina, for example, explained how she could not tolerate the violence any longer and fought back: "*Yo pase de todo tipo de violencia domestica.* [I experienced all types of domestic violence.] I was at the point that I wanted to kill him. One day I even stuck a fork in his arm." Delfina also fought back. Her boyfriend had gotten drunk one night and grabbed her by her neck. She described to our ethnographer Juanita how she had punched him, grabbed all his clothes, and put the clothes in a bag. Delfina explained disdainfully, "Fuck that shit, no man is ever gonna hit me, so I hit him back and didn't see him in days." Almost invariably, these defensive attempts were unsuccessful in halting the onslaught of slaps, punches, and worse for any noticeable length of time, and they often resulted in an escalation of the violence.

Sometimes, the women resorted to violence as a way of retaliating for the emotional abuse and betrayal that they endured. Narcisa recounted how she took revenge on her partner:

JUANITA: What happened with the guy you married? What was his name?

NARCISA: His name was Raul Sanchez. I got married to him in 2000. *Fue por interés.* [It was out of convenience.] After I married him I found out he was using drugs and was also an alcoholic. Later on I found out that he had killed his first wife and had been in prison for fifteen years. *En ves de ser una luna de miel, fue luna de hiel.* [Instead of a honeymoon it was a moon of bitterness.] He would call me Sylvia instead of my name. *El me daño la mente. Un día yo le metí una pela. Le esparate la boca.* [He ruined my mind. One day I beat him up. I broke his mouth.]

JUANITA: Why did you beat him up?

NARCISA: *Porque metió mano con un hombre, con un pato.* [Because he got involved with a man, with a gay man.] I have been divorced from him a year now. *A mi me van pasando cosas que yo me quedo boba. Yo sola no puedo batállame.* [Things have happened to me that I stay baffled. I can't battle alone.]

Even if the symptoms of severe mental illness may have predisposed the women to become involved in a relationship that was or became abusive, there remains the question of why they remained, despite the emotional pain and physical injury that they suffered. Many of the women simply did not have the cognitive or emotional wherewithal to leave, specifically because of their mental illness. Lalia, for example, who had been repeatedly raped and beaten during her marriage, likely did not have the ability to formulate a plan of action or to visualize the future. Her schizophrenia remained continuously in the foreground of her existence, plaguing her with hallucinations and depriving her of coherent thought and speech, despite her attempts to adhere faithfully to her prescribed medication regimen. She had never completed high school and spoke only Spanish, limiting her ability both to seek help to remedy her situation and to support herself and her children even if she had been able to conceive of leaving.[16]

Some of the women may have remained with their violent partners because of what has been referred to as traumatic bonding, whereby the power imbalance that characterizes a relationship is magnified over time, so that the batterer's sense of power and control increases and, concomitantly, the subjugated partner's sense of self-worth decreases, resulting in increased dependency on the batterer.[17] In Osana's case, it was not until she was confronted with the very real threat of death that she could muster sufficient courage to leave, despite her sense of failure and ineptitude. She explained how it was that she had remained with Jesus for so long, despite the agony and suffering:

> In reality, it has not been easy. Then you start analyzing your situation. Thinking about what day he started loving me. Back then I didn't talk about my past. The beatings I got. I started seeing myself in situations . . . People don't know what they get themselves into until things happened. It's hard to get out of that situation. By then you are already hurt, abused, and depressive. You have multiple conditions in your head like broken nose and fractures. You also have emotional abuse, and that is worse than physical abuse. Locked up in a bedroom, you, twenty-four hours. You can't come out if I'm not with you. He used to tell me my male friends were looking at me. He asked me if I liked that. He said someone saw you with a guy. You know he accused me of things he did. I just realized that two or three years ago when I woke up, and I thank God I never had a child from him.

Many of the women had been sexually or physically abused or both during childhood, or had witnessed violence in their homes while they were growing up. They may, as a consequence, have come to believe that this type of interaction represents the norm. Their relatively limited education and financial resources may have constrained their opportunities and limited their abilities to conceive of alternative ways of relating and resolving conflict, while their status as a minority within the larger white-dominated society may have resulted in their further devaluation and marginalization.[18] Indeed, all of these circumstances may interact in complex ways to predispose an individual to later victimization.[19] Sexually or physically abused minority children

> experience betrayal when they discover that someone on whom they were vitally dependent has caused them, or wishes to cause them, harm. . . . Sexual development and relationship skills may be shaped in inappropriate and interpersonally dysfunctional ways. Survivors may feel stigmatized, different, tarnished, spoiled. They learn to keep secrets,

> which violates a person's ability to be congruent. . . . Powerlessness becomes part of a pattern of relating when children feel that they are not in control of their bodies and their lives. . . . The awareness of racism, of being treated differently in a negative way, simply because of ethnicity, creates a feeling of a lack of safety; the world is not a good place. Children of color end up feeling less than good, second class, in our society. . . . These behavioral and emotional effects are similar to those of sexual victimization but are due to traumatic experiences because one is an ethnic minority.[20]

Maria, for example, had left her sexually abusive father and negligent mother at the age of thirteen for a relationship with a thirty-eight-year-old man who she thought would protect her. Instead, she was pregnant by the age of fourteen and had two children by the age of sixteen. She explained to Juanita during a visit to Maria's apartment,

> He was an alcoholic and still is to this day. *El iba por dos o tres dias bebiendo.* [He would leave for two or three days drinking.] I always had the kids with me, day and night. So I had no break with the children, so I would be sleepy and tired all the time. My husband came home from work, took a bath and got dressed, and left to the bar with his friends to drink. Emergencies happened with the children, and he would not be around due to his drinking. One day the baby got sick, I was in the ER all night. He came in after being gone for two days. When he didn't see us in the house he became angry. He thought we had left him because of his drinking problem. I showed him the ER papers and I asked him, "*Y tu a donde carajo estabas tu?*" [And where the fuck were you?]

Maria remained with her husband for seventeen years despite the constant beatings, believing that this was the ways things were supposed to be.

The answer as to why many of the women remained in abusive relationships may rest not only on this constellation of personal circumstances but also on the cultural expectations of both the male and female partners in the script that they created together.[21] *Machismo*, often portrayed negatively and stereotypically by the media as encompassing the dominance and subjugation of women, sexual freedom, and alcohol consumption, also encompasses positive qualities of family responsibility and honor.[22] Nevertheless, some *machista* males may enact only the more negative aspects of this quality and attempt to prove their masculinity and establish their power by controlling their female partners.[23] Men may equate male sexuality with sexual relations, penetration, their own sexual satisfaction, male dominance and control in relationships, male control over condom use, having multiple sexual encounters with multiple female partners, and a lack of concern for their sexual partner.[24] These attitudes may negatively affect the couple's ability to communicate about sex and to reduce their risk of sexually transmitted infections.[25] (It is important to note that while these attitudes and behaviors are encompassed within the concept of machismo, they are not unique to Latino culture. Indeed, many dimensions of this conceptualization of manhood and masculinity are reflected across diverse cultures.[26])

The male partner's enactment of machismo in this manner may be reinforced through the female partner's enactment of *hembrismo* and *marianismo.* Often referred to as the female counterpart of machismo, the concept of *hembrismo* encompasses qualities of strength, perseverance, and action to improve families. *Marianismo*, the "myth of martyrdom," stresses the importance of family privacy (such that personal issues are not discussed with others from outside the home), motherhood, maternal self-sacrifice for the children's benefit, and the preservation of family and marriage.[27] This construction of the woman's role has been continually reinforced by both the enunciated dogma of the Catholic Church and the failure of the legal system to protect women from retributive action by their partners.[28]

The concept of *familismo*, or loyalty to the family, may also serve to discourage women from seeking help to address the violence.[29] A *mujer buena* (good woman) would not abandon her man or discuss with people outside of the home the emotional or physical violence that pervades every moment of her life and threatens to destroy her.[30] Consequently, Latinas may be less likely than others to label behavior as abuse, believing that *debe aguantar* (she must endure).[31] Puerto Ricans, in particular, may be more approving of intimate partner violence and may be more likely to view violent conflict as the natural consequence of having violated traditional gender norms.[32] There is also evidence to suggest that Puerto Rican women who are more traditional in their sex role behavior may be more susceptible to depression, which may further compromise their ability to leave an abusive relationship.[33] As a result, perhaps, of the congruence of personal, familial, and cultural factors, Puerto Rican women experience higher rates of partner violence compared to other Latin American subgroups in the United States.[34]

Cassandra, for example, stayed with her partner despite his infidelity, despite his threats, despite his physical abuse, because he was the father of her children and it was her duty to do so. As she shared her frustration with her situation with our ethnographer Isa, she explained,

> *Como lo amo, lo odio*. [I love him like I hate him.] He is a son of a bitch. . . . He is the father of my kids. I care for him, I feel for him sometimes, but he is jealous. . . . That son of a bitch looks at women when they are dressed fresh, then look at me, motherfucker. I'm tired, Isa. [*Cassandra raises her voice*.] I'm tired of this shit, who does he think he is? I've been sick and he doesn't help me here.

Cassandra was not only a mujer buena but a "good bitch," as she had sarcastically called herself in responding to her partner, Christian. She continued, despite everything, to "clean, wash clothes, and always have dinner ready when he gets home from work."

5

Critical Others

Tu sabes que yo no cuento con mi familia.
[You know that I don't count on my family.]
—Suelita

Family of Origin

It is not difficult to understand why so many of the women experienced conflict and even violence in their romantic relationships. Many of them had experienced instability and trauma as children, and, as is common in such circumstances, these factors had led to their development of a poor self-concept, extraordinarily low self-esteem, and a distortion in their construction of relational schemas.[1] The convergence of these effects laid the groundwork for both later victimization in adulthood and a heightened risk of contracting HIV infection.[2]

Katia, you may recall, had been given up by her mother after Katia's life was threatened by her mother's boyfriend. Like most people, and as a normal part of development, Katia developed her sense of herself (self-concept) based on her evaluation of the feedback that she received from other people and on the values and expectations of others in society that she had integrated into her sense of self.[3] She developed her self-esteem from the value that others attributed to her, particularly those who were significant figures in her life, such as her parents and other family members.[4] Not surprisingly, Katia never felt valued as a child because her mother had not valued her. And not only had her mother abandoned her in favor of the boyfriend who had tried to kill her, but her grandmother also had rejected her, not understanding, or perhaps not caring, that Katia's bed-wetting was the only way that Katia could, as a child, deal with overwhelming feelings of sadness, despair, and anxiety.

Katia's feelings of hopelessness and unworthiness persisted into adulthood. A child's self-concept doesn't change easily; each person has a need to reduce ambiguity as quickly as possible (cognitive urgency) and to maintain cognitive closure (cognitive permanence).[5] Katia continued to think of herself as a failure because of the consistent negative feedback that she had received from others throughout her life, as well as the absence of other, more positive experiences.[6] As a consequence, she could not perceive her own successes and sought out circumstances and relationships that would reinforce the image that she already had of herself as worthless, unsuccessful, undeserving, unloved, and unlovable. When her emotional pain became too great, she tried to take her own life. After yet another suicide attempt, Katia explained to her psychiatrist that she had taken a bottle of pills "because I was homeless and my mom was not talking to me. My three sisters hate me." Katia's mother told one of our interviewers, "[Katia] always has problems. She gets mad at anything. . . . She has given me headaches since fifteen years old. She always comes around. She has had problems with her sisters and my sister because of her attitude."

Like Katia, Isabella had also been rejected by her birth family. Isabella, diagnosed with major depression, was thirty-eight years old when she first enrolled in the study. She had been born in Puerto Rico to a mother who had not wanted her and who had walked out of the hospital, leaving her infant daughter behind. A nurse had known of a woman with two boys who desperately wanted to adopt a baby girl and contacted her. That woman talked to Isabella's birth parents, who agreed that the woman and her husband could adopt Isabella. However, when it came time to sign the adoption papers, Isabella's parents refused to sign, even though they still did not want their child.

Isabella remained with her "adoptive" family and did not see her birth family again for eleven years. Her birth parents reappeared then and requested that they be able to take Isabella to the U.S. mainland for a short visit to meet her brothers and sisters there. However, once on the mainland, her birth parents refused to allow Isabella to return home to Puerto Rico and her family there. After a prolonged court battle, Isabella was finally returned to her "adoptive" parents, who she considered to be her real family. She had suffered during the few years that she had spent with her biological family in the United States; her biological father and older brother had sexually abused her on a regular basis, and her biological mother had done nothing to intervene, proclaiming only that she loved her little girl Isabella. When Isabella spoke to our team about the recent death of her birth father and the request by her birth mother that she pay her respects, she exclaimed angrily, "My father's body will rot before I go to the services."

Other women had grown up living in terror of their mothers, who themselves were mentally ill. Laurita's mother, Barbara, had been diagnosed with schizophrenia. As an adult, Laurita had little contact with her mother, after Barbara's then-partner and the grandfather of Laurita's daughters raped one of Laurita's daughters and Barbara castigated the injured child for bringing the incident to Laurita's attention. The grandchildren described Laurita's mother as "evil."

Many of the women had been sexually or physically abused as children by fathers, uncles, brothers, and family "friends." Research suggests that there is an extremely high prevalence of childhood sexual and physical abuse among individuals with severe mental illness. Between 43 and 52 percent of women with severe mental illness have reported being the victims of childhood sexual abuse, compared with 13 to 32 percent of women in the general population. In addition, between 33 and 52 percent of severely mentally ill women indicate that they were physically abused as children, compared with 20 to 21 percent of women in the general population.[7] Osana recounted the abuse she suffered at the hands of her brothers and her older sister, and her mother's punishment in response to her disclosure:

> I had three sisters and three brothers. Andrea was the youngest and was a sick child so my parents took her everywhere. The oldest sister, Lorena, would make the younger siblings have sex with each other. I had sex with my brothers when I was little. I was in first grade and was four or five years [old]. The situation has bothered me for years. I used to feel guilty. I blocked out a lot of things but still remember a lot of things that happened. I told my mom but she did not believe me. When I tried telling my mom she beat me with an aluminum bat. Lorena was twelve years old when all of this happened. My brothers and sisters never talked about the sex. My other brother is in Puerto Rico and has been using drugs for years. Lorena was raped by our uncle when younger.

It is not surprising that Lorena, as a victim of childhood sexual abuse herself, forced her younger siblings to have sex with each other. Children who have been sexually traumatized often become sexually aggressive themselves and victimize younger children because of the confusion around sexual norms and boundaries resulting from their own abuse. Their actions may also be an attempt to compensate for the powerlessness that they felt as victims of sexual abuse.[8] As a result of the abuse, the children are unable to feel the emotional and physical safety that is so critical to a child's development.[9] Childhood abuse is associated with later physical abuse, homelessness, depression, substance abuse, lower levels of self-esteem, and multiple physical health problems during adulthood, circumstances common to the women in our study who had been abused as children.[10]

The unease, insecurity, and distress that many of the women experienced as young children may have been magnified by their migration to the U.S. mainland from Puerto Rico. More than three-quarters of the women who participated in our study had migrated as children, adolescents, or women from Puerto Rico to urban areas of the mainland, a move that required significant adjustment. Like many other Latin American migrants to the U.S. mainland, many of the participants and their families had left Puerto Rico in search of better economic opportunities, only to find, in many cases, that the skills and relatively minimal levels of education possessed by the family breadwinners were of little use as the urban economies declined and jobs requiring unskilled labor became increasingly scarce.[11] The economics of daily living were more difficult than the migrants had initially anticipated.

Those who migrated as adult women had often left Puerto Rico feeling betrayed in love or fearing violence from their partners there. They frequently came to the mainland with their children in tow. The immediate consequence of the women's migration was an increase in the demands placed upon their time and energy to care for their children, attend to household tasks, and secure and maintain employment. This new urban environment lacked the sense of cohesion and familiarity that they had enjoyed in Puerto Rico. The migrating women also missed the emotional support that they may have had from their families in Puerto Rico and, because of the multiplicity of demands placed on them, could not provide their children with the level of attention that had previously been available to them through an extended family and social network in their place of origin. The relative absence of others in their new environments with whom they could communicate in Spanish further reduced their sense of connectedness. It is likely that many of the women and children experienced, to varying degrees, a sense of alienation, aloneness, and sadness, commonly associated with what has come to be known as "culture shock."

Although culture shock is often thought to be temporary and relatively benign in nature, its symptoms may actually be significant and its effects lasting. Culture shock "is precipitated by the anxiety that results from losing all familiar signs and symbols of social intercourse. These signs are the thousand and one ways in which we orient ourselves to the situations of daily life: when to shake hands, when and how to be gracious and appropriate . . . when to accept invitations, how to take statements seriously."[12] As a result, individuals may experience feelings of inadequacy, vulnerability, anger, resentment, and irritability, and find that they are unable to solve even simple problems because of their lack of familiarity with the new environment. They may lack self-confidence and have a tendency to blame others for any difficulties.

Katia, for example, never really felt at home in Cleveland. She often spoke wistfully about the days when she lived in Puerto Rico, reminiscing about the house that she had rented there and all of the places and parties she had gone to with friends. Katia even claimed, probably inaccurately in view of what we knew about her mental illness history and her other stories, that she had never become angry during all of her years of living in Puerto Rico and was only depressed because she was no longer there. Zamara, too, had never really adjusted to life on the mainland. She said she had hated Pennsylvania, where she had lived before moving to Ohio, and now was unhappy in Ohio. When our ethnographer Isa asked Zamara why she felt this way during a shadowing occasion at her home, Zamara explained, with sadness in her voice, "Things are different in Puerto Rico. . . . I feel lonely and lost. . . . It's hard when I am away from my family in a place where I don't speak the language." Isa indicated in her field notes, "Zamara seemed very depressed during this visit. Towards the end of the visit she was smiling because her parents were coming to visit her from Puerto Rico."

Moving On

The rejection, abandonment, and neglect that many of the women had endured as children continued to plague them in their adult lives. The majority of those to whom the women turned for assistance, counsel, and guidance—their "critical others"—were frequently no healthier mentally than the women themselves and in some cases were even less stable. Almost one-half of the individuals to whom the women turned for assistance with decision making were themselves mentally ill, almost one-quarter abused substances, and fully one-quarter of these critical others physically abused the study participant (Table 5.1). One participant, for example, continued to interact with her very mentally ill parent and had extensive contact with her boyfriend's two sisters, who were also severely mentally ill (Figure 5.1). Reflecting an all-too-common pattern, the women's romantic partners were often similar to the people who had abused them as children, and their abusive relationships mirrored the abuse they had experienced as children.[13] Yries said of her twin sister, Jimena, who had been diagnosed with bipolar disorder, "When she meets somebody good she don't know what to do."

Often, the dysfunctionality that was so evident in a participant's family of origin during childhood persisted into her adulthood. Maria's mother seemed to burst with pride in speaking about her daughter's social skills but also seemed to be in competition with her daughter for friends:

> She has been married twice. She has three girls and a boy that I know of. She had twelve siblings. Three are dead and nine alive. She has a brother and older brother in jail. Her kids are married. They have kids. She even has grandkids. She has four kids and they have kids and also married. The family has parties. She is close to them. I sometimes go when I can. At the beginning I didn't visit my family too much because I was ill. We share a lot and we are united. They are always together. Like rice and beans, that's how they are. She has a lot of friends. My friends are her friends. She has stolen all my friends. All my friends are her friends. They always ask me about her. Sometimes I don't know my friends are her friends. She steals all my friends. [*Laughing*] She has always been sociable. Ever since she was in my belly. That girl talks to everyone. She used to escape from me to be with her friends. I thought she didn't have friends but she did everywhere. She was always sassy. A sassy girl.

Frequently, it seemed that a woman's romantic partner or parent or adult child forgot that the woman was a person with a disease and approached her, instead, as a disease. As an example, a woman's husband or adult child might view her not as an individual with a diagnosis of

Table 5.1. Mental and emotional characteristics of critical others

	Relationship to study participant											
	Romantic or sexual (n = 23)		Parent (n = 7)		Child (n = 13)		Other family (n = 5)		Friend (n = 4)		Total (n = 52)	
Characteristic	No.	%	No.	%	No.	%	No.	%	No.	%	No.	%
Severe mental illness	8	34.8	4	57.1	6	46.2	4	80.0	0	0.0	22	42.3
Substance use	7	30.4	0	0.0	4	30.8	1	20.0	0	0.0	12	23.1
Physically abuses participant	6	26.1	2	28.6	2	15.4	2	40.0	1	25.0	13	25.0
Abused by participant	6	26.1	0	0.0	3	23.1	3	60.0	0	0.0	12	23.1

Note: Totals in columns may differ from total indicated by category because some critical others had multiple characteristics (e.g., they could be severely mentally ill and also abuse substances).

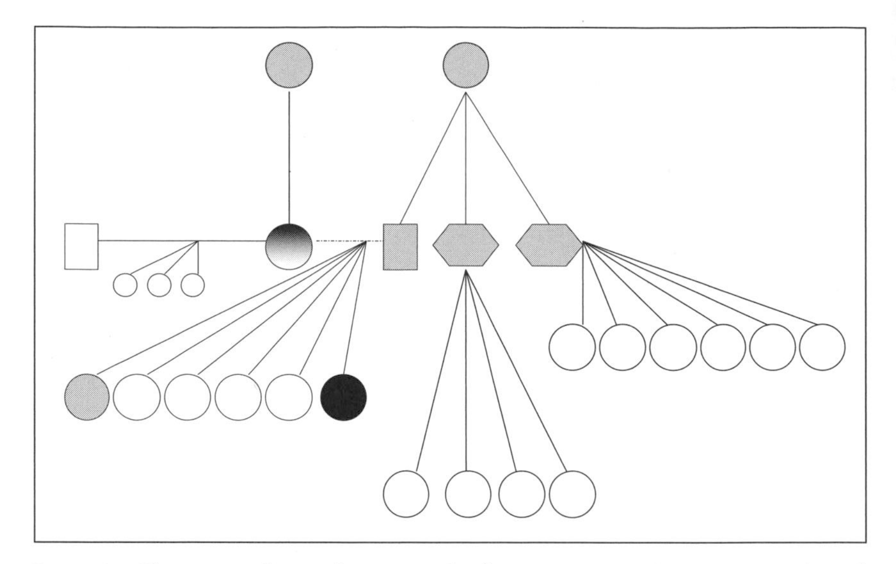

Figure 5.1. Illustration of immediate network of one participant. Participant is indicated by the semi-shaded gray circle in the center. Circles indicate parent-child relationships; hexagons indicate sibling relationships; rectangles indicate sexual or romantic relationships. Gray signifies mental illness; black signifies death. The figure does not reflect substance use disorders that exist within the network. A solid line indicates a biological or legal relationship; a dashed line indicates a nonbiological relationship or one that is not recognized legally. Younger generations appear lower in the diagram. The sex of each individual, other than the participant, is not indicated in order to preserve the participant's and her family's privacy.

schizophrenia, but instead as a *schizophrenic*, thereby disaffirming her existence and diminishing her importance. They seemed to attribute to their diagnosed family member all of the stereotypical characteristics that they had heard applied to individuals with mental illness: violent behavior, a frenzied appearance, an evil intent, and a lack of intelligence, trustworthiness, or sense of responsibility.[14] As research has shown, an erroneous belief in such a portrayal could lead one to conclude, logically enough, that the diagnosed family member was to be feared because of her dangerousness, prevented from making important decisions because of her irresponsibility, and not cared for because of her lack of intelligence.[15] Dayanara, for example, said of her mother, Elena, who had been diagnosed with schizophrenia, "Well, her face starts to change. She looks at you evil and her eyes get big and real red. Especially if she drinks. Then it gets real bad. The demon comes out of her. My mother is crazy."

The diagnosis of mental illness becomes, in essence, a "mark," or stigma.[16] In response to this mark, people may socially distance themselves from the mentally ill person—that is, set the individual apart, cease their "normal" conversations with him or her, and begin to isolate and marginalize the person.[17] The "marked" individual may, as a consequence, experience feelings of rejection, loneliness, and depression, and redefine himself or herself in order to conform to the definition that is inherent in others' treatment of the person.[18] As an example, a woman might experience even worsening self-esteem because she internalizes others' poor opinion of her and her capabilities.[19] Adalia confided to Isa her worries about her family's response to her diagnosis:

ISA: Does your family know you are on medication?
ADALIA: Yeah, they know.
ISA: How did it feel when the doctor told you [that] you were depressed?
ADALIA: I got nervous.
ISA: Why?
ADALIA: I thought it was something big, I worried.
ISA: Why did you worry?
ADALIA: Because people thought I was crazy.

We were struck by the courage that Adalia demonstrated in pursuing treatment for her mental illness, despite her concerns about her family's reaction. Many people in Adalia's situation—relatively poor and with little education—might not have pursued mental health care in the face of a potentially negative family response.[20]

Frequently, individuals will try to avoid people's reactions to their diagnosis of a mental illness by keeping it secret.[21] Yadra, for instance, never fully revealed the extent of her illness to her romantic partner. She explained to Juanita, one of the study ethnographers,

> Now it is mainly at nighttime that my head starts running and I start having the flashbacks of all the bad stuff that has happened to me. *Todo es malo. Por eso yo no quiero que el viva conmigo. Pa que no se de cuenta.* [Everything is bad. That is why I do not want to live with him. I don't want him to notice.] Because I am embarrassed. He knows that I suffer from depression and take medications but he does not completely know about my condition and my past. I also do not

> want to tell him because I don't want him to think that he is superior to me.

And, in an attempt to avoid the possibility of unpleasant interactions with and demeaning responses by others, a person may isolate herself even further.[22] Dayanara noticed that her mother seemed to keep herself apart from other people after she was diagnosed with schizophrenia: "She probably thinks people are going to look at her different. Like weird? Yeah, she might think that. I don't know if it's the depression [that is] why she doesn't talk to people. I really don't know because she wasn't like that."

A number of the participants recognized the problematic aspects of their then-current living situations and chose to isolate themselves in order to minimize their involvement, knowing that such isolation was potentially detrimental to their mental health. In an example of the proverbial "damned if you do, damned if you don't," Elena, who was in recovery from substance use, explained why she self-isolated when her daughter's boyfriend was around: "Hector has his friends coming over every day smoking weed and getting high. I was in my room all the time. I was in my room all the time and that's not good for me. I just stay in my room. When I come out, I say hi, how are you, and go back in."

Sometimes, family members limited the individual's social contacts with others, believing that they are not capable of relationships because of their mental illness diagnosis. Regardless of whether the isolation is self- or other-imposed, it may be particularly harmful for individuals who have been victimized by abusive partners. As Elena realized, isolation may exacerbate symptoms of depression and feelings of alienation. Often, abusive partners isolate their victims; increasing the abused person's social support system may be a necessary and critical step toward recovery from the abuse, the redevelopment of trust in the environment, and the reconstruction of self-esteem.[23]

Natalia had had a representative payee appointed by the Social Security Administration to manage her money; her case worker there believed that Natalia was too ill to make rational decisions about the use of her limited funds and, accordingly, had appointed Natalia's friend Josefina, who Natalia regarded as a mother, to fulfill those responsibilities. As such, Josefina was obligated to use Natalia's funds for Natalia's benefit. This status gave Josefina almost complete control over Natalia's access to funds and any activities that required funding.

But Josefina extended her control even beyond this. She did not isolate Natalia from all others, but often intervened to limit or prohibit altogether Natalia's contact with specific individuals. It was difficult to determine whether Josefina's pronouncements and unilateral decision making undermined Natalia's efforts to expand her horizons or protected her from probable harm, whether Josefina's extensive involvement with the details of Natalia's life reflected an underlying belief about the ineptitude of mentally ill people or a realistic appraisal and concomitant concern for someone with limited abilities. We wondered whether Josefina's constant advice was not actually harming what little self-esteem Natalia possessed. As an example, Josefina had discouraged Natalia from pursuing her romantic interest in a particular man:

NATALIA: My mom [representative payee] told me I am not ready to have a relationship with him because he was high functioning.
ISA: What did that mean?
NATALIA: Someone who doesn't have schizophrenia or bipolar.
ISA: Did you ask your mom what that meant?
NATALIA: My mother said that I need to be with someone at my level.
ISA: What level was that?
NATALIA: At a low-functioning level.
ISA: What does that mean?
NATALIA: I have mental problems so that [not being low functioning] means I have my own place and pay the bills. . . .
ISA: Do you think you are low functioning?
NATALIA: I don't know. . . . My mom wants me to be with a guy named Dante from church. . . . Dante is low functioning like me and my mom likes Dante.
ISA: Do you like Dante?
NATALIA: No. I am mad because my mom said I am acting like I was in heat. . . . It was not funny.
ISA: What did your mom mean?
NATALIA: My mom said I am still recovering and should not be in a relationship with anybody.

Natalia is particularly low functioning, not only as a result of the effects of her schizophrenia but also because of what appears to be a developmental disability. In an interview with the ethnographer, Josefina described Natalia as a "little girl hidden in a big body. Very sweet, innocent. When she [is] angry she becomes this grown adult. She can lash out with harsh words. . . . Then becomes apologetic. Recognizes she was wrong. Goes back to childhood feelings of guilt from childhood rape. Trust everybody. Innocent stage of not recognizing danger. Because of lack of love." Our own interactions with Natalia convinced us that she was, indeed, childlike and vulnerable, eager for attention from anyone, no matter what the ultimate emotional or physical cost.

Onlookers, and even some mental health care providers, might characterize Josefina's involvement in Natalia's affairs as excessive, believing that such an intense level of involvement effectively stifles the attempts of a severely mentally ill individual to achieve a greater degree of independence and possibly leads to rehospitalization.[24] Others might suggest that this level of involvement reflects an over-involvement in the life of a mentally ill person and is symptomatic of pop psychology's diagnosis of codependency.[25]

Natalia was, in fact, rehospitalized several times during the course of the study. And although Natalia chafed under Josefina's supervision and prohibition against the pursuit of her romantic interest, it appeared to us that Josefina's involvement also provided Natalia with the sense of belonging and being cared for that she so desperately sought, a need that frequently remains unmet among individuals with severe mental illness.[26] For many individuals of ethnic minority status who have been diagnosed with a mental illness, this level of involvement might provide them with a sense of family cohesion and help to decrease their mental illness symptoms and diminish their level of emotional distress, rather than being detrimental to their prognosis.[27]

The "mark" that the women bore was sometimes compounded by other features of their lives.[28] Communication between Elena and her daughter, Dayanara, had diminished following Elena's diagnosis of schizophrenia, but their relationship became even more complicated after Dayanara realized that her mother preferred women rather than men as her sexual and romantic partners. Although Dayanara claimed to have accepted her mother's sexual orientation, she made it clear that her acceptance had its limits:

ISA: Did you ever have a stepmom?
DAYANARA: Like living with us?
ISA: Yes.
DAYANARA: No, I would not go for that.
ISA: Why? And what about if it makes her [Elena] feel happy?

DAYANARA: I would feel uncomfortable having a woman live with us. I mean, they can kiss in front of me, but that's about it.

Dayanara indicated that she had never shared with her mother her own discomfort at the thought of her mother's lover residing with them, but it is likely that Elena sensed her daughter's uneasiness because she never suggested that her partner move in with them, despite the years that they had been together as a couple.

Jimena, too, appeared to be marked by both her mental illness and her sexual orientation. Jimena's twin sister, Yries, remarked to one of the study ethnographers that Jimena "don't barely got any friends." She attributed the absence of friends in Jimena's life to both her sexual orientation and her temper, which was a symptom of her bipolar disorder. The sense of alienation that Jimena felt may well have been related to her diminishing morale, if past research findings in other studies are to be believed.[29]

Teodora depended on her family members but often felt discouraged, hurt, and angered by the way they spoke to her. Of her brother, she said, "He calls me a fucking bitch. Everyone in this house is mean. They call me names. My mom is something else too." Vyna had similar experiences with her family, who seemed not to understand that her moods had nothing to do with them but were often a function of the highs and lows of her depression and frustrated her as much as they did her family. Vyna had written in her journal, "My mother hates me. . . . [She said] I was an ungrateful bitch, a beast, and that I was a monster." The hostile and negatively charged emotional responses that were directed toward Teodora and Vyna are known as expressed emotion. High expressed emotion has been found consistently to lead to a worse prognosis among individuals diagnosed with schizophrenia.[30]

Many of the women felt betrayed by the very people on whom they depended for emotional support. Yries recounted to one of the ethnographers how she had been betrayed by her sister, whom she thought she should have been able to trust:

YRIES: I was homesick; [the city where I was] was so fucking small that you can pretty much walk everywhere, you walk ten minutes and you are in downtown. Karl was always out and about with his friends, leaving me alone, so I came back to Cleveland in three weeks. We continued talking after that. He wanted to come to Cleveland and stayed with me for a while but I kicked him out when I saw he touched [my sister]. Then he said he had slept with [my sister], but she denied it. I left him alone, I was with nobody for a minute.

JUANITA: Tell me about the issues with your sister. She has dated the same guys you have, did you ever have an understanding about it, did you talk about it?

YRIES: It has happened. I'd tell [my sister] if her date tries to touch me, but she still stays with them. Once we went to a psychic and [my sister] confessed she had slept with two of my boyfriends. I cared but I didn't care, that's still my sister, but I told her, I don't trust her. I keep my eyes open.

JUANITA: How do you feel about it?

YRIES: I'm supposed to be trusting her, she's my sister, I shouldn't be doing that, not trusting her.

Osana also felt betrayed by her friend, who had reported her for working while she was receiving housing assistance. Osana had been trying to save money, to have something in the bank to cover unexpected emergencies, instead of surviving from one month's assistance check to the next. She explained to one of the ethnographers what had transpired, but did not want the conversation taped. The ethnographer noted,

> She said she doesn't tell a lot of people she has Section 8 because she had a bad experience once. I asked her what happened, and she said one of her friends called the SSI office and told them she was working. Osana said she could not believe her friend did that because she helped her out with groceries and gave her clothes. I asked her why her friend did that, and she said she was jealous of her. Osana said she didn't expect that from her.

The betrayal that Honoria felt from her husband, Alfredo, bordered on abuse. Frustrated with her situation, she cried out,

> Your husband doesn't use drugs, right? He doesn't wake up every day looking . . . you have clothes with the price tags in the clothes. You have shoes in your closet. You buy shoes and clothes and food. You buy things to clean your house, your husband doesn't take them to sell them. He wakes up and is sick [needs to inject drugs], he takes them back to the store and gets the money back. Takes the things you bought

together? . . . He doesn't sell [them], right? I buy food and he goes and sells it for two bags of drugs. I get WIC and he sells it for two dollars at the store. He goes to the store, gets money for the coupons. . . . Do you have that kind of life? Right, you go to the store, you buy your things, happy, then get home. You don't have to worry about someone returning your things. You have perfumes, right? I don't have perfume because he returns everything back or sells it. He don't got no clothes. I don't have that much clothes. You understand what I'm saying. Groceries, he sells them and when I have a baby, is he going to stay hungry because he will sell the baby formula? . . . I tell you because of what you are doing. I don't tell my problems to anyone because nobody can do nothing for me, you know, no one.

Ties That Bind

Many of the women were emotionally close to the individual they had designated as their critical other, at least in the sense of sharing the intimate details of their lives with them; however, relatively few could count on their critical other for positive emotional support. In some cases, the lack of support may have been due to the limitations of the critical other, caused by their own mental illness symptoms or substance use, or by the demands associated with maintaining employment, nurturing their own romantic relationships, and caring for other children. In other cases, the critical other may have felt overwhelmed by the emotional energy required to attend to the needs of an adult whose behavior may have seemed bizarre or felt abusive. (As Table 5.1 indicates, almost one-quarter of the individuals designated as critical others were abused by the study participant.)

It was hard to know, sometimes, where emotional support and caring ended and overprotectiveness began. Yadra's mother, Maritza, for example, had tried to warn her daughter about the disaster that she foresaw in her daughter's relationship with her boyfriend. She had seen that Yadra's partner was involved with multiple women; indeed, he had been kicked out of a rehab program for his heroin addiction when he was discovered having sex with one of the women there. Maritza tried to protect her daughter, she explained, because she saw how Yadra had changed as her depression deepened over time: "She would not put up with so much [before], and she would make better decisions. When depressed she locks herself up.

She would have better friends, better relationships with her sisters. Yadra is intelligent. If it were not because of the depression she would be able to work like she used to."

If it were not for Josefina's presence, it is likely that one of Natalia's many failed suicide attempts might have succeeded. Despite all of Josefina's criticisms of Natalia, it was Josefina, after all, who interceded and brought Natalia to the hospital, after enlisting the aid of their pastor, when Natalia's auditory hallucinations returned and her paranoia escalated:

> She knew that something was bothering me, and I just started crying and she said, Natalia what is it? And I said, it's the voices again, mom. She said, now you know where you need to go. I want you to go to the hospital and be evaluated. I just cried. She said, don't cry. You will be all right. You have been through this before. But it's hard. . . . I feel like I am an outsider. . . . I started hearing the voices so my mom, Josefina, told me to go to the hospital 'cause my [surrogate] sister knows, Coraly knows I wasn't eating, I was isolating, I was crying, I wasn't talking. I just wasn't being me so she told [my roommate] Celia and Celia told the pastor and the pastor said I had to go to the hospital. Then Sunday morning they brought me here.

It could not have been easy for the families and friends of the participants to make themselves available emotionally on a consistent basis.[31] Many of the women experienced frequent and dramatic mood swings, which among some of the women were exacerbated in frequency and intensity by alcohol and drug use. Not surprisingly, family members often find it particularly difficult to devote time and energy to relatives with co-occurring mental illness and substance use disorders because of the associated increased frequency of criminal behavior, verbal outbursts, and physical violence.[32]

While Jesusita suffered from the symptoms of her severe depression, her husband, Eleazar, felt that he also bore his own suffering with her illness:

> She is cold. She is not affectionate. She has always been that way. . . . I would like for her to be different. We are never together. When we are home she is always doing her own thing. At times I feel unsatisfied sexually with Jesusita because of her coldness. When I look for her in a sexual way she almost always turns me away because of tiredness,

> headaches, or makes something up. I feel rejected because she does not want to have relations. . . . I initiate the acts.

Eleazar acknowledged that, despite Jesusita's apparent distancing from him, they still engaged in sexual relations together an average of two to three times each week. It was her coldness and emotional distance that caused him pain.

Of all the critical others identified by study participants, friends seemed to be the most emotionally supportive and present the fewest problems of their own. Unlike family members, who research has found often expect something from their mentally ill relative in exchange for their investment of time, energy, or money in their ill relative's well-being, friends appear to have relatively few expectations of a reciprocal exchange for their efforts.[33] Also, friends, more so than family members, seemed to recognize the importance to mental health of maintaining an emotional connection with others and remaining active. For example, Isabella's friend Javier Cristobal said of her, "When depressed, she wants to be by herself. Now she is not like that. . . . Going out more often, I think, has helped her a lot. She is not the same person that was always in the house. Now she goes out and distracts her mind."

It was an entirely different story when it came to providing support in the form of material assistance. Relationships with critical others, be they parents, adult children, friends, or more distant family members, might be cold, dysfunctional, abusive, or even violent. Nevertheless, the vast majority of the participants could find physical shelter in the home of their critical other, reducing drastically the occasions on which they might otherwise have found themselves homeless and on the street. This provision of only one type of support by members of our participants' social networks is a common characteristic of the networks of severely mentally ill people. It stands in sharp contrast to the provision of multiple forms of support (termed "multiplexity") often available from social network members to individuals without severe mental illness.[34]

All of our participants' critical others were themselves Latino, although they were not all Puerto Rican. It is possible that the critical others willingly provided this form of assistance to demonstrate to the participant *respeto*, a cultural value that "addresses the need to maintain and defend one's personal integrity and that of others, and to allow for face-saving strategies whenever conflict or disagreements evolve."[35] By providing shelter to a woman who would otherwise be homeless and even more vulnerable, the critical other defends his or her own personal integrity, as well as that of the ill individual.

The cultural value of *familismo*, too, likely played a role in critical others' decision to help and the nature of the help that they provided. Familismo, or familism, has been called one of the most important culture-specific values among Latinos and particularly among Puerto Ricans. It has been defined as a cultural value that includes a strong identification and attachment of individuals with their nuclear and extended families, including "adopted" friends and family members, and strong feelings of loyalty, reciprocity, and solidarity among members of the same family.[36] It can be thought of as the ties that bind family members together, whether family of birth or, as is common in Puerto Rican culture, chosen family, much as a shoe is bound together by its laces to maintain its usefulness, however new or worn, polished or tired-looking the shoe may be.[37] The value of familismo may be manifested structurally, through reference to the spatial and social boundaries "within which behaviors occur and attitudes acquire meaning and are delineated by the presence or absence of nuclear and extended family members";[38] attitudinally, through the beliefs and attitudes regarding the family with respect to feelings of loyalty, solidarity, and reciprocity; and behaviorally, through the actions associated with those feelings.[39] The attitudinal component is particularly important because it serves as the foundation for the family members' interaction, determining the extent to which the needs of the family and family members are to be placed before individual interests, the extent of interconnectedness between family members, the extent of family reciprocity in times of need, and the behaviors that are expected in order to maintain and defend the family's integrity.[40] The Latino family may play a singularly critical protective role because of these strong ties and high levels of mutual loyalty, solidarity, reliance, and trust.[41]

This may explain why, for instance, severely mentally ill individuals who are Latino are less likely to be homeless than individuals from various other ethnic groups.[42] The provision of this tangible form of support has wider implications than only shelter; individuals' ability to secure some form of shelter is an important factor in their care, as homeless individuals with severe mental illness are more likely to need emergency care and psychiatric hospitalization.[43] Stable housing may also reduce severely mentally ill individuals' risk of violent revictimization, with its own consequent risks of retraumatization, unplanned pregnancy, and sexually transmitted infections, including HIV.[44]

6

Motherhood

Si mis hijos no hubieran llegado yo me suicide.
[If my kids wouldn't have arrived, I would have committed suicide.] . . . I am here for my kids. I dedicate myself to them. So I have a meaning to live. It has always been that way. *Mi autoestima esta por el piso.* [My self-esteem is on the floor.] Only my kids keep me going.
—Yadra

Mis hijos son mi vida. [My children are my life.]
—Typical saying in Puerto Rico

Among women with severe mental illness, motherhood may fulfill a particularly important role in their lives, serving as an affirmation of their importance and providing a mechanism for the expression of feeling and the fulfillment of an important social role.[1] This is not surprising, since parenthood provides many individuals with a way to demonstrate creativity and nurturing.[2] Parenting that is perceived as successful may boost an individual's self-esteem and feelings of self-worth and competence. Accordingly, women with severe mental illness may begin their childbearing early and have multiple children.[3]

Motherhood is a particularly important role in the context of Puerto Rican culture.[4] Although the males of the family are to be respected and often hold significant power, it is the mothers who are perceived as the glue that binds the family together.[5] U.S.-born Latinas often begin their childbearing years at a younger age compared to females of other racial/ethnic groups in the United States and tend to have a higher fertility rate.[6] Compared to both other Latino subgroups and non-Latinos, Puerto Rican females are more likely to begin their childbearing during their teenage years, are less likely to have an abortion, and are more likely to have a greater number of children.[7]

Historical events may have also shaped the culture's views of the importance of reproduction and motherhood. America's quest for racial purity through the legalized forcible sterilization of often unknowing women was brought to Puerto Rico, then a territory of the United States, in the 1930s.[8] With the approval of the established eugenic sterilization board, a total of ninety-seven eugenic sterilizations were performed during the years 1937 through 1950; the eugenic sterilization law remained in force until its repeal in 1960.[9] Although many voluntary sterilization procedures were performed during this same period of time, the extent to which they were truly voluntary in the larger context of limited family planning options remains contested to this day.[10]

Family planning efforts instituted in Puerto Rico were, and continue to be, similarly controversial, viewed by opponents of these programs as an American effort to erase the island's population and by proponents as a step toward modernization, the reduction or elimination of island poverty, and the improvement of maternal and child health.[11] However, because of the limited availability of contraception and contraceptive advice, a great number of women turned to contraceptive field trials as a means of obtaining these products. Many of the products used in these trials were ineffective and substandard, leaving women feeling that the products were worthless. Researchers later conducting Puerto Rico–based field trials of birth control pills often dismissed women's complaints about the pills' side effects as unscientific, psychosomatic in nature, and the result of women's "emotional superactivity."[12] The extent to which women opted for "voluntary" sterilization under such circumstances remains uncertain.

Whether the participants of our study were knowledgeable about these historical details is unclear, although at least a few had heard vague murmurings about the use of Puerto Rican women as guinea pigs in birth control experiments.[13] Regardless of the reasons, motherhood and children played a critical role in the lives of a great majority of the women in our study. Almost all of the women (90.6 percent) had at least one child, and some had as many as eight.

Even those women who already had several children often expressed a wish for more. Adalia, who already had four children, had lost them to her ex-husband and to social services because she had been unable to care for them as a result of her severe depression. Frustrated, she had had her tubes tied (a tubal ligation). Now, she missed her babies and was trying to save enough money to have surgery to untie her tubes.

Many of the women encountered enormous practical difficulties in their role as mothers. As is not uncommon among mothers with severe mental illness, many of the women faced parenthood as what has euphemistically come to be known as "single heads of household," with all of the attendant issues: lower income levels, limited employment opportunities, and, in many cases, victimization by partners. Delfina, diagnosed with bipolar disorder and only twenty-four years old at the time of her enrollment into the study, explained the circumstances surrounding the birth of her son: "I got pregnant when I was fifteen years old. . . . When I got pregnant he wanted me to have an abortion. We were kids. He doesn't pay child support. I lived in a shelter for the whole nine months when I was pregnant. He said the baby wasn't his. We even had a paternity test. It came out Jonathon was 99.9 percent her father."

Honoria, whose emotional swings associated with her bipolar disorder were poorly controlled, felt overwhelmed with her responsibilities as a single parent:

> HONORIA: [*Shaking her head from side to side and crying*] Now I have a baby. I feel depressed, so depressed. [Alfredo, the baby's father] is not going to help me with her.
>
> ISA: Why? Where is he?
>
> HONORIA: In the streets, you know. The same thing.
>
> ISA: Do you think he'll help you with the baby?
>
> HONORIA: [*Opens her eyes*] No! Him? No.
>
> ISA: He won't help you feed her at nighttime?
>
> HONORIA: Him? Get up? No way. I'm tired. I haven't sleep in three days.
>
> ISA: Who was there when you had the baby? Your mom?
>
> HONORIA: Yes, she was there. Alfredo [*laughs*] he almost fainted. He saw the baby coming out and kept saying, "Look, Honoria, look!" I told him I can't see. He asked me again, Isa. Look, he is crazy. I could not see.

Despite their difficulties, both Delfina and Honoria, like many women with severe mental illness, lived with the fear that they might lose their children to child protective services because of their mental illness.[14]

Several of the women had become pregnant without understanding quite how it had happened. Although Zamara was already twenty-five at the time that she enrolled in the study, we learned over time through successive shadowing occasions that she had little knowledge of either her own anatomy or the process of pregnancy. Her first pregnancy, she explained, had ended in a miscarriage: "I didn't know I was pregnant. I was in the back of [my place of employment] putting some things away. The delivery truck delivered some boxes. I picked up a heavy box. Then I felt a sharp pain and I started bleeding everywhere. I went to the bathroom. When I got up there was a ball of blood in the toilet."

Zamara became pregnant again, believing that she could not become pregnant with her boyfriend: "I never used protection because I didn't think I was going to get pregnant by Alexander. I thought he could not have any children because he is thirty-something and doesn't have children." This time she decided to have an abortion, although she had always felt that abortion was morally wrong. Isa, the ethnographer, asked her whether she had considered giving the baby up for adoption. She said that she had, but had rejected that option because she had been drinking and was concerned about both the child and her ability to care for the child: "I can't take care of myself let alone a child. I worry that child may be sick and be an alcoholic." Despite the ever-present symptoms of her depression and the difficulties she experienced trying to control those symptoms, despite her own lack of understanding about how she could have become pregnant, and despite her drinking, Zamara was concerned for the welfare of her unborn child. Our ethnographer accompanied Zamara to the abortion clinic, at Zamara's request, and waited for her in the reception area while Zamara underwent the procedure. Zamara felt physically exhausted and emotionally drained afterward, commenting only, "I wish I had an angel to talk to."

Pia, also, had not understood the connection between intercourse and pregnancy. She had left home at the age of sixteen in an attempt to escape the sexual abuse she had been enduring. Pia explained, "I did not know anything about birth control when I was growing up. My mother never spoke to me about sex or birth control. I learned about birth control on my own and by getting pregnant several times." A devout Catholic, Pia had decided against an abortion with any of her pregnancies. Now in her early forties, she had seven children. She had had her tubes tied after her last child in an effort to prevent any additional pregnancies.

Some of the women had become mothers at an early age, perhaps because of their own lack of understanding about either contraception or the complexities of life with a child. Being a teenage mother can bring its own set of problems. In addition to the increased stress and constrained educational and occupational opportunities now facing the mother, there are heightened risks for the baby, including low birth weight and an increased risk of neonatal mortality.[15] Legal problems could also demand the mother's attention, as Imelda, who became pregnant with her first child at the age of sixteen or so, discovered:

> ISA: Why didn't [your boyfriend] give his last name to the baby, Imelda?
>
> IMELDA: Because I was not eighteen, you know. . . . He could have gotten in trouble. But now I can't get [the baby's] social security number or birth certificate until he puts his last name. That is going to take about a week or two. If he doesn't want to put his last name I'll find someone else.
>
> ISA: You'll find someone else to give the baby a last name?
>
> IMELDA: Yes.
>
> ISA: Why do you want to give him someone's last name?
>
> IMELDA: I don't want him to have my name. I want him to have a father, you know, but he doesn't want to do it. He doesn't want to be a father. The only one that wants to be a father is [my friend] Ricardo and my boyfriend.
>
> ISA: And does he [the baby's father] call you?
>
> IMELDA: From time to time. He asks for the baby but he keeps on talking about me.
>
> ISA: What does he say?
>
> IMELDA: I tell him I don't want to talk to him anymore. I don't want anything to do with that man.
>
> ISA: Really?
>
> IMELDA: I don't want to do anything with that man and if I don't use the last name, what can I do? I would have to put my last name.

Though many were still barely middle-aged at the time of their participation in the study, they were already grandmothers. Their grandchildren gave them even more joy, it seemed, than had their own children, despite the difficulties associated with caring for them, and gave the women a purpose for living. Despite their poverty, their mental illness, their conflicted relationships, they often went to great lengths to make life pleasant for their grandchildren. Elena, for example, was only forty-two years old when we first met with her, and already had seven children and a number of grandchildren. She had been diagnosed with schizophrenia and often felt depressed with her situation:

> ELENA: I'm depressed. First thing I do when I get up in the morning is smoke. I don't care anymore. I don't care if I live or die.
> ISA: I understand what you are saying. So, when you are feeling that way is health important?
> ELENA: No, nothing is. *A mi la vida no me importa.* [Life is not important to me.] I always knew there was something wrong. . . . My granddaughter is what keeps me—
> ISA: Keeps you from?
> ELENA: She keeps me from killing myself.
> ISA: Do you think of killing yourself often?
> ELENA: Yes. All the time, but she needs me and no one is there for her so she keeps me wanting to be with her. I have one boring life.

Child rearing can be particularly difficult for women with severe mental illness because of the convergence of multiple factors: economic hardship; limited education or employment opportunities; unstable housing situations; absent or abusive partners; disorganization, negativity, anxiety, and social isolation associated with their mental illness; poor parenting role models; a lack of understanding of and difficulty negotiating the child's developmental phases; and the adverse effects of their own childhood experiences of neglect, abuse, and parental substance use or psychopathology.[16] Nevertheless, despite these often daunting circumstances, the majority of the women did their best to raise their children.

Much of their effort focused on providing, as best as they could, shelter, clothing, and food to their children. Isabella and her husband, Christophe, for example, had struggled to save enough money to move their children into a new home in a less poverty-stricken and crime-ridden neighborhood. They spent a tremendous number of hours beautifying the rooms that were to be their children's. Isabella proudly showed their daughter's room to Juanita, the ethnographer. They had painted the room white with specks of light pink and furnished it with a white day bed and dresser, a perfect setting for their little princess. The two boys were to have bedrooms on the second floor, where Isabella's husband had knocked down the walls so that their rooms would be "a decent size" for two growing boys, as Isabella explained.

Lalia typified many of the women in the study in her concern for her children. Lalia asked that our ethnographer Isa accompany her to one of the local nonprofit organizations where she could buy toys and clothes for her children. Lalia dressed up for the shopping expedition, donning a white tank top and black slacks, with a small black purse and white tennis shoes to accessorize her outfit. Once there, Lalia gleefully ran through the store, sifting through the clothing on the racks to find just the right outfit for her son.

At times, the women's efforts to provide for their children were frustrated by people they had trusted. Ida, only eighteen years old at the time that she enrolled in the study and suffering from major depression, was already mother to a young child. She had been able to obtain a stroller and some clothing for him from a nonprofit agency. When our ethnographer Isa visited her at her home, however, she learned that Ida's former boyfriend had stolen all of the baby's furniture and some of his clothing and had sold it all for drug money. Ida had started to think about the need for a restraining order against him and was searching once again for baby furniture and clothing at various nonprofit agencies.

Like many mothers everywhere, they tried to teach their children the basic skills of everyday living. Osana recounted an episode that had occurred with her boyfriend's daughter and how it had provided the impetus for her to have yet another discussion with her children about the need for cleanliness: "The other day Leonardo's daughter stained my bathroom carpet. When I saw it, I was upset. She is messy. She was on her period and didn't flush the toilet. I sat with them and told them about personal hygiene. I tell them to set the table at dinnertime and after dinner to clean their own area."

Many of the women also tried to impart to their children the wisdom that they had garnered from their own life experiences. Suelita, for example, explained to the ethnographer Juanita how she both counseled her daughter and warned her to forget about having a boyfriend in her efforts to protect her daughter from sexual risk:

JUANITA: How about with your kids, do you talk to them about sex?

SUELITA: Oh yeah, especially my daughter. She asks questions about stuff, too. Like she has asked me about feminine products. She has large breasts already for her age. I always tell my daughter to concentrate in her studies. *Ellos saben lo que es bueno y lo que es malo*. [They know what is good and what is bad.]

JUANITA: What kinds of stuff have you told them?

SUELITA: I have told them to let me know if anyone ever touches them inappropriately. I feel comfortable talking to them about drugs and sex. *Le estoy diciendo to lo que es bueno y lo que es malo.* [I am telling them all that is good and all that is bad.] The kids are always fighting with me about smoking 'cause they know that is bad for me. They even know the difference between what is marijuana and what is not. A lot of that stuff they learn at school. They come home talking about that stuff.

JUANITA: What kinds of stuff are they learning at school?

SUELITA: About STDs and drugs. I do worry about my daughter getting to [that] age. By her body you can tell she will be well developed and that scares me. *Mi hija ha estado media malcria ultimamente pero yo la endereso. Yo le digo a ella que su novio es la correa.* [My daughter has been a bit misbehaved lately, but I am going to straighten her out. I tell her that her boyfriend is (my) belt.]

Mireya, too, attempted to provide guidance and counsel to her children as they matured into adolescence. She explained to the ethnographer Isa:

MIREYA: My sister started giving her kids birth control pills young. She is liberal, she let her [daughter] have boyfriends and they come to visit her at the house. I tell my son I'm going to buy him condoms. I tell him he needs to be careful where he sticks his dick.

ISA: What does he say?

MIREYA: He laughs. I tell him the difference of using and not using a condom.

ISA: What do you think is the difference?

MIREYA: Staying without diseases.

ISA: How about the girls?

MIREYA: It depends on how fast they are. Girls can be fast.

ISA: Fast in what?

MIREYA: In developing, and what worries me is my son doing drugs. He always asks me if I trust him. He tells me he won't do drugs because his uncle does it and he sees how he is. I asked him if he plays with himself and he laughed.

ISA: How would you feel if he told you he is having sex right now. Would you get mad?

MIREYA: I would get mad. . . . It depends who he's having sex with.

ISA: What do you mean?

MIREYA: If the girl is fast or older. I think he plays with himself. I want to be the one in charge of talking to my son about sex.

ISA: Why you?

MIREYA: Because I want to know everything, and I know what to tell him.

Many of the women, though, had difficulty establishing close ties with their children or recognizing parent-child boundaries and appropriate methods of discipline. Problematic parenting, including negative and tense parent-child interactions and difficulty establishing parent-child attachment, is not uncommon among women with lower psychological functioning;[17] worse maternal psychological functioning may be linked to the mother's own experiences of childhood abuse.[18]

Commonly, the women had difficulty recognizing where the boundary might exist between parent and child in their respective roles, or even understanding that such a boundary should exist. Celestina, who described her relationship with her friend Maria as so close that they could be *primas* (cousins), recounted how Maria had involved her young daughter in her most recent suicide attempt:

> I only know that Maria was talking to [her boyfriend] on the phone and they were arguing, and when she hung up, she started screaming and yelling and throwing things to the wall, she went crazy, and then is when she got the pills and asked *la nena* [the child] to bring her water to take the pills. She took the pills in front of the girl, that's so wrong. So the girl called me crying and scared, so *me desesperé, yo estaba como loca* [I became desperate, I was going crazy], you know I suffer from nerves, so when *la nena me dijo eso* [the girl told me that], I got agitated. I told her, "*mamita, llama a la ambulancia*" [baby, call the ambulance], but she didn't want to because she said her mother told her not to call or that she would spank her. She was so scared, but she didn't want to call the ambulance and she kept asking me what to do. I was with my husband so he saw me so upset that he called the ambulance. When Maria saw the ambulance she thought I called it and she got angry with me and she said not to call her anymore, that she didn't want to see me anymore. And that hurts my feelings, because all I wanted was to help her, I never wanted to cause her harm or problems, I wanted to save her life, because I didn't know if the pills she took were already in her system, she could

> die. But now she thinks I wanted social services to take her daughter. How can she think I would want that? I love this girl as my own, I would never want anybody to take the girl from her, all I wanted was to help her.

Boundary issues were also evident in Maria's interactions with her son. Maria explained to our ethnographer Isa how she regretted the overtures that she had made to her son while she was under the influence of cocaine:

> MARIA: I'm doing a moral inventory.
> ISA: What does that consist of?
> MARIA: Everything bad and hurtful things I did. I told my son sorry for telling him I wanted to have sex with him while I was drunk.
> ISA: Do you remember saying that?
> MARIA: Yes, I remember everything. When I told my son I wanted to have sex with him I was drunk and I used cocaine. I told him that.

A number of the women were clearly frustrated when their children failed to obey them or made what appeared to them to be unreasonable demands. Laura, the mother of three children, had been diagnosed with bipolar disorder. She had been a victim of childhood abuse and, more recently, partner violence. Consistent with what is seen in many individuals with bipolar disorder, she had once used cocaine, had been a "cutter," and had attempted suicide.[19] She and her children lived in relative poverty, attempting to subsist on her income from social security disability, which she received on the basis of her mental illness diagnosis. Laura, like the vast majority of parents in the United States, used corporal punishment as a means of disciplining her children.[20] Laura described how she had used corporal punishment with her children: "When I get depressed I don't deal with anyone. When they start to depress me [*looking at her children*] my blood gets hot. I hit them with my punches. I broke [my daughter's] mouth and if she keeps on, I'll do it again. I'm just like that. They know that. When I feel like that I feel my body shaking." The memory of their mother's past physical and verbal outbursts was often sufficient incentive for Laura's children to refrain from engaging yet again in behavior that could provoke another such outburst.

It was not uncommon for the women to use corporal punishment to discipline their children for displaying *una falta de respeto* (a lack of respect). Elena, for example, explained to our ethnographer Isa how and why she had slapped her eighteen-year-old daughter Dayanara:

> ELENA: The other day I smacked Dayanara.
> ISA: You hit her?
> ELENA: Yeah.
> ISA: Oh! Oh! What happened and when was this?
> ELENA: Last week, and she wanted Hector to stay over and I said no. She called me a son of a bitch so I slapped her. Look, I have a bruise (pointing to wrist). I hit her by her eyebrow where she has that earring. That area is red. She covered herself with her hands so I didn't get to hit her good.
> ISA: Did she hit you back?
> ELENA: Oh no. She would have hit me back, I would have really hit her like a man.

It was clear that Elena believed that her physical response to Dayanara's verbal insult and disrespect was reasonable, justified, and warranted. The contradiction apparent to us in the use of physical force with a grown child to retaliate for verbal disrespect was not similarly apparent to Elena.

There exists considerable disagreement as to the boundary between physical abuse and "legitimate" corporal punishment.[21] Corporal punishment has been judged to be appropriate when the physical force is used to cause "a child to experience pain, but not injury, [and is] for the purpose of correction or control of the child's behavior."[22] We encountered a number of situations in which we, as a team, felt compelled to evaluate the need to report a particular research participant to child protective services because of suspected child abuse. We were not under any legal obligation to do so because of the certificate of confidentiality that we had obtained from the National Institute of Mental Health. Nevertheless, we felt an ethical obligation to report child abuse and had advised participants as part of the informed consent process that we would do so if we encountered it, in order to avert any further injury to the child. We struggled to understand whether the behavior that we sometimes witnessed was truly abusive or merely offensive to our own middle-class standards of child rearing. In those few situations that may have bordered on abuse, we weighed our ethical obligation to maintain the participant's confidentiality and our ethical obligation to protect the child, frequently consulting with psychiatrists and other mental health professionals in the process.

Invariably, we found that these situations were already under investigation by county authorities, sometimes as the result of a teacher's report, a probation officer's referral, or the report of a neighbor. Sabrina, for example, recounted to our ethnographer how both of her children had been taken from her after her oldest child reported being hit by her:

> JUANITA: How are your kids doing?
> SABRINA: Fine, I guess. My daughter was living with me from December till April but she had to leave.
> JUANITA: Why?
> SABRINA: *Por que yo le di.* [Because I hit her.] And she called the social worker. The social worker came and took Melanie and then went to the school of my youngest daughter and took her away as well. That was terrible for me because I would never hit my youngest. The whole time she was gone I would just play video games and go dancing and that was it. When we went to court, the judge asked the social worker why she took the youngest and she did not have a response.

Published literature suggests that nonabusive Latina mothers have a greater number of warm and caring relatives within their social networks and have more extensive contact with their relatives than do abusive Latina mothers.[23] The family contexts in which we encountered situations that could have potentially been characterized as abusive seemed no less dense and no less caring than those of our other participants.

Like many mothers, the women frequently interacted with significant figures in their children's lives. Mireya, for example, had been telephoned by her son's elementary school teacher, who explained that her son had urinated on himself yet again and asked her to please come down to the school and bring him a clean set of clothing. Elena had received a phone call from her daughter Dayanara's probation counselor, asking her to remind Dayanara that she was to present herself for drug testing again; routine drug testing following the birth of Dayanara's child had revealed that Dayanara was using marijuana and the baby had been removed immediately from her custody by the county.

Many of the women were actively involved with the mental health care system not only because of their own illness but also because of their children's difficulties. Children of mentally ill parents appear to be at increased risk of psychiatric disorders,[24] interpersonal difficulties, and behavioral problems.[25] Consequently, despite their own sometimes severe limitations, the women were frequently called upon to act as advocates and case managers for their challenged and challenging children, a role that is common to families with a mentally ill member.[26] Mendi, for example, often juggled appointments with her son's teacher, doctor, and school counselor. After he ran out of the house with a knife, child protective services also became involved, as she explained to our ethnographer Anastasia:

MENDI: Since I don't have money, I'm in a bad mood and I fight with him [my son] for silly things. Then *el nene me pone mala* [the child gets me mad.]

ANASTASIA: What does he do?

MENDI: He's hyper, he's too much. I'm trying to get pills for him to see if that calms him down.

ANASTASIA: Wow, he's five, right?

MENDI: Yes, but he's been like that since he learned how to walk. *Me ha estado dando candela desde los dos años.* [He's been giving me fire since he was two.] He fights with his sister. She's quiet but he gets her upset, so then they fight. That also upsets me, when I see them fighting, *me pone mala* [it makes me sick].

ANASTASIA: Wow. So you said you want him to get medication for that?

MENDI: Yes, I've been talking to his doctor, but I need his teacher to write something saying he needs it, because he's very young and the doctor can't prescribe it without more information about his behavior in school.

ANASTASIA: I see. He sees a doctor only or he also has a counselor or social worker?

MENDI: Yes, he has a counselor, because *él ya me sacó cuchillos* [he already got out knives].

ANASTASIA: Knives, wow, what did he do with knives?

MENDI: He went in the kitchen and got a knife and went running outside, so I was running after him, but I was afraid that if I got on him he could fall and hurt himself with the knife, so I had to wait to get it back. So, they called social services on me.

ANASTASIA: Social services? You mean child protective services? Why?

MENDI: Yeah, children services, because I said I couldn't get the knife from him, but they closed the case. They came and saw they had their clothes and food and that the house was clean. I told them he was hyper and that's why he has his doctor and the counselor. Yeah, *el no me hace caso* [he doesn't obey me]. I have to be on him twenty-four hours, there's no rest with him, only when he's in school I get a break, poor teacher. He can't see me calm, he has to start something to get me upset. People tell me he needs pills.

ANASTASIA: So what does the counselor recommend?

MENDI: She tells me *que añoñe al que pierde la pelea* [to pamper the one that loses the fight].

ANASTASIA: What does it mean?

MENDI: Because they are always fighting, so she tells me to comfort the one that loses the fight, so the other one is not going to want to fight more, but that is hurting my son, because he thinks I care more for my daughter and he screams at me, "I hate you!" He has even said he wants to kill himself, that he doesn't love me.

Children of mothers with a mental illness are more likely to have a mental illness themselves, which is likely attributable in many cases to the combined effects of genetics and environment.[27] A number of our participants' children were diagnosed with various disorders, including depression, attention deficit hyperactivity disorder, and conduct disorder. Catalina knew that there was something wrong with her son, Nestor, who had repeated the ninth grade three times. Despite Catalina's difficulties brought on by her own depression, she had pleaded repeatedly with his school counselors to conduct a formal assessment in the hope that they could identify what was troubling her son. After her many appeals continued to be ignored, she finally retained an attorney to argue with the school for her. Catalina explained to our ethnographer Juanita how she worried about Nestor constantly:

CATALINA: I am concerned about Nestor. If it wasn't for that pill, he wouldn't get up. . . . Look what Nestor did to me the other day, he was hiding in that corner all covered up when I got home from work. When I saw that I started trembling, and this shameless son of mine gave me a scare. *El va muy mal. Lo veo enfocando un camino que no me gusta.* [Real bad. I see him leading to a path that I do not like.]

JUANITA: Are you getting any help from the school?

CATALINA: Those people don't know what they are doing. I don't know how they claim to help kids with special needs because they really don't help at all.

JUANITA: Catalina, what has Nestor been diagnosed with?

CATALINA: *El tiene un monton de cosas.* [He has a bunch of stuff.] He has attention deficit disorder and anxiety.

Despite Catalina's attempts to intervene and obtain help for her son, he tried to kill himself. Home after five days in the hospital following his suicide attempt, Nestor explained why he wanted to die:

NESTOR: *Mi mama te cuenta mis loqueras?* [Does my mom tell you about my craziness?]

JUANITA: Well, what are you referring to?

NESTOR: Well, yesterday I had an incident. I tried to hang myself with a phone cord. I was hanging there for one hour and a half before my mom found me. I tried to pull down on the cord but I would not die. It was *Papa Dios* [Father God] [*pointing to the sky*].

JUANITA: Why did you want to die?

NESTOR: Because of women problems.

JUANITA: What do you mean?

NESTOR: I keep running into women *que solo quieren chingar* [who only want to fuck] and that is it. This has happened to me with at least seven women. The last one I was with, we were having sex all the time and she claimed that she loved me and wanted to marry me. Then the next day she acted differently with me. Yesterday I left her a long message insulting her and calling her every name in the book. She called me back crying. We were both crying on the phone. She told me that we would get together today and talk things over.

For others in our study, whatever intervention may have been possible to help their mentally ill child was too little, too late. Marisa's son Kenneth, only ten years old, had succeeded in his most recent of many attempts to end his life. She talked about his suicide but did not want the conversation to be recorded. The ethnographers' notes reveal what Marisa recounted:

> She told us that she has been depressed for four days now. She said she has just been thinking of Kenneth's death. Isa asked if she missed him. She said yes. I asked her how it was that Kenneth died. She said, "*Se me holco*" [He hanged himself]. Marisa said that he was always taking GI Joe men and tying them up by the neck. She said that he hanged himself with a military belt. She said that she thought he was just playing but that the military belt has a strong lock and he could not get himself out in time and hung from the bunk bed with the belt around his neck. I asked her where was she. She was in the basement doing laundry and after a while she asked, "*A donde esta Kenneth?*" [Where is Kenneth?] She said that her son Benedicto was the one that found him and that has really affected him. She said that the boys had seen her boyfriend at the time be abusive to her and that has also affected them. I asked her where was that boyfriend now. She said he was in jail and she hopes he stays there. She said that she blames him for Kenneth's death.

Marisa remembered Kenneth with a photo of him and her other two sons. She comforted herself with a large gold cross that she had taken from Kenneth's hand after the wake.

7

Adrift

Navigating Systems and Bureaucracies

It is a waste of time talking to my social worker because Puerto Rican families don't do some of the things she suggested.
—Mireya

Accessing Services

Numerous reports have documented alarming deficiencies in the availability and provision of mental health services to those in need of them. As an example, among individuals with depressive disorders who are seen in general medical practices nationally, only about 50 percent are actually recognized by their providers as being depressed, and only one-half of them receive appropriate treatment; this means that 75 percent receive either no care or inadequate care.[1] Studies have consistently shown that Latinos are much less likely than whites to receive appropriate care for mental illness.[2] And, among those who are depressed, Latino patients are less likely than non-Latino white and African American patients to receive specialty care for their depression.[3] These deficiencies are even more pronounced among those who are poor or uninsured.[4] The women in this study met with numerous obstacles in their attempts to access both mental health care and other needed services. Even when they were able to obtain services, the adequacy of those services was sometimes questionable.

As an example, one of the study ethnographers became concerned during a shadowing episode that Yadra, who suffered from major depression, might be on the verge of a suicide attempt. She obtained Yadra's permission to call the hotline for the crisis unit, hoping that someone there could intervene appropriately since Yadra's mental health care provider was inaccessible. The ethnographer's notes reveal the futility of that effort: "I called the mobile crisis unit from her [Yadra's] house. The worker that answered said that since she [Yadra] has a mental health provider and it is still during business hours, she needed to contact them to make the assessment on her. He said their services would be on an after-hours basis if she would not be able to get in touch with the office of her mental health provider."

The only option remaining to Yadra, like many other severely mentally ill individuals with poor access to outpatient care, was a visit to the emergency department of the local hospital.[5] This was not the first time Yadra had had such difficulty contacting her provider. The ethnographer's notes had documented other, similar instances: "She [Yadra] said that she has called her social worker over eight times and she has not returned her calls. She said that she could no longer leave any more messages because it says that her mailbox is full."

The long waiting time to be seen at the emergency department of local hospitals frequently complicated efforts to obtain care. Longer waits meant taking the younger children along, and that could mean spending more money on transportation to get there. Leaving them at home meant that they would be unsupervised for a longer period of time, and that could mean more issues with child protective services. Marisa, diagnosed with schizophrenia, had three young children at home. She prevailed upon our ethnographer Isa to take her to the emergency department to be seen for the severe abdominal pain that she had been having for several weeks already. She was finally able to go, she explained, because her father was visiting her from out of state and could watch the children while she was at the hospital. By the time Marisa was seen at the hospital, almost four hours had passed since her arrival there. It was some time later that she was informed that she had a bladder infection and that she was able to obtain the medications necessary for its treatment.

Stigma

Even after accessing services, clients with severe mental illness may continue to encounter barriers. One might think—and even expect—that professionals in the mental health field would approach their clients non-judgmentally, understanding the embarrassment, the fear, and the isolation that often accompany symptoms of mental illness, even before a formal diagnosis is made by a mental health professional. Even mental health care professionals, however, have been found to be stigmatizing of their clients, using pejorative terms to describe them or their symptoms, disbelieving their physical complaints, ridiculing their mental illness symptoms, and devaluing their efforts to achieve a more stable existence.[6] In one study of mental health service consumers, more than one-quarter of the respondents reported having been the focus of stigmatizing behavior from their mental health providers.[7] Sometimes, providers may also stigmatize the client's entire family (stigma by association) and blame the family members for the client's mental illness.[8]

Like a number of the women in our study, Lalia encountered such attitudes from the first moment she set foot in the door of the agency where she was to receive mental health care. Lalia, born in Puerto Rico and almost monolingual in Spanish, had been diagnosed with schizophrenia. Even after conquering all of the logistical challenges that she faced to get to her appointments—transportation, child care, fatigue—she met with yet another obstacle: the receptionist at the mental health agency. Lalia explained,

> She thinks she is an executive there. I have seen the way she is with other people. People think that because you have a mental illness that you are crazy. There is a lot of discrimination against the mentally ill. I can't believe they keep her there. She is the first contact person. She should be pleasant. *Yo estoy enferma pero no loca.* [I may be ill but I am not crazy.] There are worse things than having a mental illness, like prostitutes and drug addicts.

Other study participants had similarly unpleasant interactions at the agencies from which they received care. One commented about the receptionist at her provider's office, "This old woman is so rude and nasty, I don't know how she can work there if she treats people like that." Yet another study participant offered the following remark about an office assistant: "You know that she is supposed to call the patients to remind them of their appointments. She never calls me. I told [my therapist] she never calls me. . . . If her job or her life is so bad she should go work somewhere else. One already feels bad when you go there. She makes you feel worse."

Like many individuals who endure the stigmatizing attitudes of their mental health care providers, Osana's experiences with her social worker left her feeling that she had to be guarded in what she revealed.[9] Osana related her social worker's reaction to her confidences: "I can tell when I tell her things she opens her eyes like if it's evil. She has never paid me a visit, never. Linda looks at me and thinks everything is a sin." We do not know whether Osana's perception of her social worker's responses was an accurate one. Our ethnographers accompanied Osana on several occasions to these appointments, but it is impossible to know whether their presence at these sessions somehow modified the dynamic between Osana and her social worker. However, other research suggests that providers may be ambivalent about sexual expression among women with severe mental illness, and that ambivalence may erect a barrier to the women's efforts to obtain complete care.[10] The inability to be frank with her social worker may well have compromised the quality of care that Osana was able to receive.

The Provider-Patient Alliance

The establishment of a therapeutic alliance between provider and patient may be critical to the patient's adherence to medication, continuation in treatment, and sense of empowerment to manage his or her illness. The concept of a therapeutic alliance, derived from the Greek word *therapeuein*, meaning to serve, and the Latin word *alligare*, meaning to bind, refers to the establishment of a relationship based on trust, empathy, respect, agreement, and collaboration.[11] That said, the interactions between many of the women and their mental health providers fell far short of anything that could reasonably be said to resemble an alliance.

Some of the participants faced a basic and obvious barrier to the establishment of a therapeutic alliance with their therapist: their provider spoke only English and they spoke only Spanish or primarily Spanish and relatively limited English. For example, Lalia was unable to communicate with her provider because of the language barrier that existed between them. Evidencing both frustration and impatience with her situation, she had remarked, "In order for us to communicate, he has to have a dictionary."

The inability of the patient and provider to communicate adequately in the same language has serious implications for the accuracy of diagnosis and the quality of treatment provided. Patients who speak English as a second language have been seen as demonstrating greater levels of pathology when interviewed in English, rather than in their primary language of Spanish.[12] They may feel split off from their affective experiences and developmental issues that arose prior to their acquisition of the second language, a phenomenon known as the detachment effect.[13] Additionally, because individuals speaking in their second language may have to focus greater amounts of attention on the form of their communication, such as syntax and word selection, they may focus less on the content of their communication and, as a consequence, be more likely to intellectualize and appear less responsive.[14] It has also been suggested that individuals may be more tense when responding in their second language and, as a consequence, may be less expressive and appear more withdrawn. As a result, the therapist may misinterpret these behaviors as evidence of a lack of motivation, withdrawal, or depression.[15]

It is not surprising, then, that a number of the women felt caught in what seemed to them to be a battle between their English-speaking and Spanish-speaking mental health care providers. Yadra, for instance, commented that her English-speaking social worker "has a different diagnosis from the psychiatrist. You would think they work together." Of her psychiatrist, she said, "*El me entiende más. No se si es por que hablamos el mismo español.* [My social worker] *no me entiende.*" (He understands me better. I don't know if it is because we speak the same Spanish. [My social worker] does not understand me.)

The providers' lack of familiarity with the women's culture similarly erected a barrier to the establishment of a therapeutic alliance; more than one-half of the women indicated that cultural issues interfered in their ability to obtain adequate care (Table 7.1).[16] Lalia was frustrated by both her provider's inability to understand Spanish and his unfamiliarity with the cultural milieu in which she lived: "I am being seen by [a provider], but he is American and does not really understand my language. Sometimes I tell him things and he has to keep questioning me to try and understand what I am trying to say. That frustrates me."

Like the inability to communicate in the same language, a provider's lack of cultural familiarity may have serious implications with respect to the quality of his or her assessment and treatment approach. The provider may misinterpret the client's unfamiliar behavior as evidence of mental illness when it is not (known as overpathologizing bias) and erroneously diagnose the client with a mental illness. Conversely, the provider, perhaps in an attempt to be culturally sensitive, may mistakenly attribute

Table 7.1. Mental health service utilization of the study participants

	Primary language of participant								
	English (n = 7)		Spanish (n = 29)		Bilingual (n = 17)		Total (N = 53)		
Service use	**No.**	**%**	**No.**	**%**	**No.**	**%**	**No.**	**%**	**p-value**
Type of service used[a]									
Social worker	3	42.9	21	72.4	8	47.1	32	60.4	0.08
Primary care physician	3	42.9	11	37.9	7	41.2	21	39.6	1.00
Psychiatrist	2	28.6	20	69.0	9	52.9	31	58.5	0.04
In-patient hospital	1	14.3	8	27.6	4	23.5	13	24.5	0.91
Emergency department	0	0.0	5	17.2	3	17.7	8	15.1	0.75
Substance treatment	1	14.3	3	10.3	0	0.0	4	7.6	0.34
Other	2	28.6	12	41.4	7	41.2	21	39.6	0.86
None	2	28.6	1	3.5	2	11.8	5	9.4	0.11
Frequency of service use[b]									
Regularly	2	28.6	19	65.5	8	47.1	29	54.7	
Sporadically	2	28.6	2	6.9	6	35.3	10	18.9	
In crisis only	1	14.3	7	24.1	1	5.9	9	17.0	
Never or almost never	2	28.6	1	3.5	2	11.8	5	9.4	0.05
Psychiatrist language[c]									
English only	1	50.0	1	5.3	5	55.6	7	23.3	
English and Spanish	1	50.0	18	94.7	4	44.4	23	76.7	0.01

Social worker language[c]									
English only	0	0.0	3	15.0	5	71.4	8	28.6	
English and Spanish	1	100.0	17	85.0	2	28.6	20	71.4	0.01
Current medication use									
Yes	2	28.6	21	72.4	10	58.8	33	62.3	
No	5	71.4	4	13.8	7	41.1	16	30.2	
Unknown	0	0.0	4	13.8	0	0.0	4	7.6	0.02
Systemic barriers to service use[a]									
Language	1	14.3	25	86.2	1	5.9	27	50.9	<0.0001
Cultural issues	1	14.3	25	86.2	4	23.5	30	56.6	<0.0001
Stigma	0	0.0	12	41.4	7	41.2	19	35.8	0.12
Insurance	4	57.1	11	37.9	7	41.2	22	41.5	0.35
Child care	2	28.6	10	34.5	4	23.5	16	30.2	1.00
Transportation	6	85.7	16	55.2	7	41.2	29	54.7	0.13

a. Totals more than 100 percent within each language group are due to the participant's selection of multiple categories.

b. Regularly refers to services used every three months or more; sporadically refers to services used less than four times per year; crisis refers to services used only for trauma.

c. Proportion calculated based on number of individuals using service, rather than entire sample.

the client's behavior to cultural beliefs and practices when it is actually indicative of an existing mental illness (known as minimization bias) and inadvertently limit or foreclose the client's access to needed care.[17] Providers' lack of cultural familiarity may explain why Latinos are overdiagnosed with major depression and underdiagnosed with schizophrenia spectrum disorders, despite the existence of psychotic symptoms.[18]

It is possible that Lalia's provider's lack of cultural familiarity may ultimately influence her decision about whether to remain in care. Numerous studies have found that Spanish-speaking individuals in need of mental health care may be less likely to drop out of treatment if their provider is bilingual and bicultural.[19] One study involving 5,983 outpatients at a large urban hospital found that inpatients who had been matched to ethnically focused psychiatric units were more likely to follow up with treatment after they were discharged, reducing the likelihood that they would be re-admitted to the hospital.[20] The matching of patients to ethnically focused units helped to enhance their communication with and trust of their providers, thereby improving their participation in treatment.

Many of the women felt that their providers simply did not listen to them or make any attempt to understand what they were trying to communicate. Yadra expressed her frustration with her therapist: "[My therapist] tells me to think that I am safe in my space and that nothing is going to happen to me, but if it was that easy and I could control my thoughts I would not be depressed in the first place and he does not understand that. I don't feel he hears me."

Mireya, diagnosed with major depression, was also frustrated by her social worker's seeming lack of understanding of the world in which she lived. She had been brutally beaten by her ex-husband, who had been convicted and imprisoned because of his violence toward her. He had been released from prison, and Mireya was fearful that he would find her—so fearful, in fact, that she would awake startled from her sleep in the middle of the night, feeling that he had somehow entered the room and was standing alongside her bed, although he was not. One of the study ethnographers accompanied Mireya to a session with her social worker, Roberta, during which Mireya confided her fears, hoping that the social worker could provide her with some advice or guidance that would at least help to alleviate some of her anxiety. Roberta's words left Mireya feeling even more dejected than she had when she arrived. Roberta had responded to Mireya's disclosure of her fears by saying, "You are acting like a child because you let your daughter know that you are scared to see her father. You need to take control of the situation. You are the mother and you need to be able to address the situation with control. . . . The police are always available and if something happens all you need to do is call them. You don't need to be the victim. Don't allow yourself to be the victim." Roberta, it seemed, was not cognizant of the possibility that someone could be beaten or killed while waiting for the police to arrive, or maybe even as they were attempting to reach for the phone to call the police.

Melasia, who had been diagnosed with bipolar disorder and had previously injected heroin, was frustrated with her psychiatrist. She complained bitterly about his lack of attention to what *she* considered to be her problems and his preoccupation with what *he* thought should be her problems: "The doctor just wants to talk about the voices. I got more problems than just voices. I keep myself busy and try to ignore the voices. But what about the depression?"

Honoria, who had been diagnosed with bipolar disorder, was an observant Catholic and concerned about her relationship with God. She had tried to explore her questions about the larger meaning of her existence with her mental health care providers, but, as she explained to one of the study ethnographers, she found the exchange less than helpful:

HONORIA: Psychologists don't believe in God, just medication. I don't like psychiatrists too much.

ISA: How come you don't like psychiatrists?

HONORIA: I don't. They ask you a lot of questions. When you try to explain things to them, it's like they don't understand. They stay looking at you like crazy. You talk to a psychiatrist and they think you are crazy.

ISA: What does it mean to be crazy?

HONORIA: OK. You know when I went to the psychiatrist, I was looking for God. Then he started asking me what I thought was going to happen after I die.

ISA: He asked you that?

HONORIA: Yeah. He asked that. You know when you see them at the beginning.

ISA: Like the first session.

HONORIA: Yeah, he asked me why do I talk about God. I told him Christ was coming and I get scared because I can't stay here on earth and that's why I go to church. This guy looked at me like I was crazy. You know, he was looking at me weird. I was embarrassed and I can't do it anymore. I can't see a psychiatrist anymore. You tell him things about God and they only think about science. They think you are crazy.

ISA: What do you think psychiatrists are for?

HONORIA: Well, psychiatrist is there to help people. That's why God put science there, to help people. The same thing is for other doctors that make pills and so forth. Understand? Science is a part of God.

ISA: So, you think a psychiatrist's job is to give pills?

HONORIA: I don't know. I was sent to a psychiatrist. [My friend] told me there are two types of psychiatrist. One is a psychologist and the other a psychiatrist. I think the psychiatrist is for the crazy people. What do you think?

ISA: I think psychiatrists are the ones who write up the prescription for pills. I think the psychiatrist has more education and background on medicine.

HONORIA: I like to talk to the people who work with the psychiatrist. I don't know what they are called.

ISA: You mean the case managers?

HONORIA: Yeah, the social workers then.

ISA: Why do you like talking to them better?

HONORIA: Because they listen to you. They give you advice on things you can do. Understand?

ISA: Yes.

HONORIA: Let's suppose you have a problem and they listen to you and give you advice and what do to. They are like, like they help you better. They listen. The psychiatrist asks question like if you can sleep at night and if you see ghosts at nighttime. He asks if you hear voices and gives you pills. That's it.

ISA: So, you think doctors are supposed to listen to you?

HONORIA: Yeah. It's not all about giving you pills. Anyone can do that. I can do that. I can listen to you and then tell you that you need pills. Why do you think a lot of people do drugs in the street?

ISA: Why?

HONORIA: Because they have problems and find relief in the drugs.

ISA: So, what do you think is the difference between street drugs and the pills the psychiatrist gives you?

HONORIA: Both are drugs.

ISA: OK. What do you think is the difference?

HONORIA: One is prescribed and the other is illegal.

ISA: Why do you think people seek drugs in the street and not see a psychiatrist for pills?

HONORIA: I think it's more convenient to find them in the street. You have to explain a lot to the doctor and you might not get the pills but in the street you just buy them, no explanations to that motherfucker [psychiatrist].

ISA: Let me ask you another question. Do you think if it wasn't for the questions or because they look at you crazy, people would see a psychiatrist to obtain pills for their nervous condition?

HONORIA: Because of what?

ISA: OK. Suppose if the psychiatrist listened to you and he doesn't look at you crazy. Do you think people will go to them faster than going in the streets to get medicated?

HONORIA: Well, some people are on Xanax, right, which is an addictive pill like Valium, but when the doctor doesn't give them to them they look for it in the street. The pills are cheaper in the street and you don't see a doctor. The problem is that psychiatrist helps people but they have not gone through the problem the patients have. Like take for example [my husband]. The psychiatrist has not been through a situation like that or what I've been through. He gives you a medication based on what he has heard about you but he doesn't know your past, like why you can't sleep or why you have nightmares. Understand? Or where you grew up at.

ISA: He doesn't ask you any of that?

HONORIA: No, they don't ask you that. Look, if you have used drugs in the past, they won't help you because you used drugs.

In some cases, the provider's lack of respect for the client was all too obvious. The transcript of Yadra's visit to the emergency department of a local hospital, which was also attended by one of the study ethnographers, Juanita, serves as an illustration. After Juanita explained to the physician in the emergency department that she had brought Yadra there after Yadra had voiced an intent to kill herself, Yadra explained to the physician the source of her distress. The physician ignored Yadra, who was the patient, and spoke to Juanita about Yadra in the third person, and somewhat disapprovingly at that:

YADRA: My significant other is currently in a rehab program. Someone from the rehab told my sister that he recently had a baby five days ago and that he needed permission from the rehab to go and give the baby his last name.

DOCTOR: So this is over a man? Can't she see that men can come and go and they are not worth it?

JUANITA: Well, obviously she does not see it that way.

In some cases, it was clear that the mental health care provider was either unaware of or did not respect the boundaries that exist between provider and patient, and that should exist in order to protect the patient.[21] Yadra said, "All the counselors do is talk about their personal problems and don't really help the participants." Lalia, an attractive middle-aged woman, had terminated her relationship with a previous therapist because she could no longer endure his incessant flirting and sexual innuendo. Her perception of this previous therapist could not be dismissed as a part of a delusionary system; other participants complained that they, too, had experienced this same therapist's sexual advances, wondering all the while if he actually expected them to respond welcomingly to them.

The unexpected provision of material assistance by several of the providers to their clients helped to foster trust and a sense that the women were truly cared for. Elena, diagnosed with schizophrenia, had been hospitalized after she had attempted suicide yet again. She was particularly pleased that the staff had unexpectedly attended to some of her more immediate needs, as she explained to the ethnographer:

ISA: What happened that you were in the hospital?

ELENA: I got an ataque de nervios.

ISA: Really, did you start shaking or what?

ELENA: I started to shake and swear and I wanted to hurt myself. The voices again.

ISA: What were they telling you?

ELENA: To kill myself, throw myself in front of a car and jump off a bridge. I tried from the porch. I almost jumped. I wanted to hurt myself. Dayanara got me and took me to the hospital. I know throwing myself off the porch would not have killed me but I want to hurt myself and maybe I would die.

ISA: How did they treat you in the hospital?

ELENA: Good, real good. Look, they even gave me shoes [*points to feet*], clothes, and a coat. [*Opens the closet door to display a coat.*] Look, it's big on me but it's nice.

ISA: It is nice. Did they give you those tennis shoes?

ELENA: Yeah, and this pants and shirt.

ISA: That's good. I'm glad. Did you like being there?

ELENA: It was OK, but I didn't like the people who talk to the voices all the time. They talk to the voices all the time. The doctor said if I don't take care of myself I can talk to the voices too. When it gets bad people start talking back to them, they engage in conversation.

ISA: Have you even spoken back?

ELENA: One time, I told them [the voices] to leave me alone.

ISA: Did they give you medicine?

ELENA: Yeah, I have them. They treated me nice and I'm better now.

Mireya had often complained about her social worker's apparent lack of interest in her life and her general lack of understanding of Mireya's situation. However, her social worker's attempts to obtain material assistance for Mireya and her children, instead of "just talking," signified a turning point in their relationship as therapist and client:

ISA: How's it going with Roberta?

MIREYA: Roberta has changed a lot.

ISA: Oh yeah, how has she changed?

MIREYA: She is different. She signed up the kids for coats. For Christmas she will help me to get toys.[22]

Attention to such materials needs of clients receiving public mental health care would most typically fall within the province of a case manager, responsible for both the coordination of the clients' treatment and the continuity and integration of needed services, such as medication management, arrangements for suitable housing, and the management of daily activities.[23] However, Latino clients with mental illness, and especially those who are Spanish-speaking, are significantly less likely to receive such services compared to white clients.[24] This is particularly problematic, as intensive case management services may be critical to the maintenance of mental health, the avoidance of homelessness and hospitalization, and the improvement of life satisfaction.[25] In our study, only 60.4 percent of the participants received services from a social worker, and not all of the social workers assigned to them served as case managers (see Table 7.1).

Numerous factors likely account, to some degree, for the difficulties participants experienced in obtaining suitable care. First, it is possible that some or all of our participants had unrealistic, and perhaps even unreasonable, expectations of their providers with respect to the nature, intensity, and frequency of the services to be provided. In some cases, for example, the participant may have expected her social worker to provide case management services, but that social worker may have been charged with the responsibility of providing counseling services only. In other cases, the participant may have demanded counseling in addition to case management services from individuals who had neither the training nor the responsibility to provide anything other than case management services. We do not know what participants expected in this regard.

Many of the social workers, case managers, and psychiatrists working within the publicly funded mental health care system carry inordinately heavy caseloads that often include a large proportion of individuals in need of intensive and varied services. They may be overwhelmed and, in some cases, "burned out" by the sheer volume of their caseloads and the intensity of their clients' seemingly never-ending needs. As a consequence, they may be less responsive to the clients' needs or demands than would be ideal. In addition, despite their professional status, they may have little or no control of their work situations and no power to modify them unless they choose to leave the public mental health care system. The number of providers available and the programs provided are largely a function of the budgets available to each public entity at which they work. Those budgets are directly dependent on the dollars provided by the state of Ohio, which has been gradually and continuously decreasing expenditures for mental health services.[26] As the need for mental health services increases along with the increasing levels of stress among the general population caused by Ohio's deteriorating economy, the shrinking number of providers faces a growing number of clients, many of whom have increasing needs. It is not unusual, at this point in time, for providers to carry as many as fifty or sixty individuals in their caseloads, all of whom have multiple complex needs that require attention. Consequently, the providers are simply unable, within the framework of a work week, to meet their clients' needs with the optimal frequency and intensity that their clients might expect or require.

Finally, on a national level, we are facing a dire shortage of bilingual and bicultural mental health providers.[27] This is not to imply that a mental health care provider must be Latino to provide culturally sensitive and appropriate services to Latino clients. Clearly, classism, ethnocentrism, and other factors may affect the adequacy of services even between a Latino provider and a Latino client. However, regardless of the personal characteristics of the provider, he or she must be fluent in both the language and the culture of the client. In view of the shortage of such professionals nationally, and the declining dollars available in Ohio to pay them, it is not surprising that many of our participants encountered cultural and language barriers in their efforts to obtain care. And, while one can understand objectively the need to make hard decisions in the face of diminishing funds, one must question the underlying wisdom of slashing funding for mentally ill people and consider whether there may exist an underlying bias in favor of those with a louder political voice.

Better Living through Chemistry

Almost one-third of the women did not use medications indicated for their mental illness while they participated in the study (see Table 7.1) and many more used them only intermittently, a pattern that has been noted consistently among psychiatric service consumers.[28] For some of the women, this reluctance or complete refusal to adhere to medication resulted from the unwelcome side effects of the drugs. Isabella, for example, did not take her antidepressant medication according to the schedule she had been given because of the side effects. She explained why she used them only intermittently: "They make me drowsy. I take them depending on how I am feeling and if I want to sleep or not. *A veces me tomo dos o tres dependiendo si quiero dormir.* [At times I take two or three, depending on whether I want to sleep.]"

Other participants experienced other unwelcome and unpleasant side effects. Narcisa explained to our ethnographer the effects of the medication that she had been prescribed for the depression associated with her bipolar disorder:

NARCISA: The medicine that the psychiatrist was giving me was affecting me.
JUANITA: Which one?
NARCISA: Wellbutrin.

JUANITA: How was it affecting you?

NARCISA: It was irritating my ulcers and I was breaking out in cold sweats. It has also caused me weight loss.

Teodora, also diagnosed with bipolar disorder, was particularly disheartened about the side effects of her medication, as she explained to Isa, the study ethnographer:

ISA: Are you on medication?

TEODORA: I'm on Depakote 500 milligrams, Celexa in the morning, and Seroquel at night time.

ISA: Do you take your meds?

TEODORA: Not all the time because I hate medication, the feeling they give me. I get drowsy and have no control of emotions. I feel numb and have no strength.

ISA: So, the meds make you sleepy?

TEODORA: Sleepy is not the word. I get *real* sleepy. That's not a way to live.

On yet another occasion, Teodora had said of her medications: "Those pills make me feel dead like a zombie."

It is not only the side effects of the medications themselves but the consequences of these side effects as well that may dissuade individuals from adhering to their medication regimens. Side effects such as restlessness, involuntary movements, and uncontrolled speech (termed "extrapyramidal symptoms"), as well as significant weight gain, may signal to others that the individual has a mental illness. This may result in the individual's isolation by others or self-isolation in an attempt to avoid the possibility of public humiliation and embarrassment.[29]

Many new medications have been introduced during the past decade for the treatment of various mental illnesses that are equally as effective as the older ones and have fewer side effects.[30] However, they are often less available to minority patients.[31] This may be due, in part, to the limitations imposed by individuals' health insurance coverage for these expensive drugs and, in part, to physicians' belief that minority patients are less likely to follow the prescribed medication regimen.[32] Over time, however, these newer, more expensive medications may actually be more cost-effective because they may reduce the need for hospitalization.[33]

Despite their side effects, Lalia continued to take her medications, finding that she could not live without them. She described her medications and their effects to our ethnographer Juanita:

LALIA: *La trazodone son para los bajos y altos. Me achocan. Risperdal son para el desorden mental.* [Trazodone is for my highs and lows. They knock me out. Risperdal is for my mental disorder.] The thing is that I have had trazodone in my body for so long that it no longer knocks me out. Right now I am at 100 milligrams.

JUANITA: Why do you think that the doctor recommends you taking so many meds?

LALIA: I just think the doctor exaggerates with the meds. If he is not changing the meds he is playing with the dosage. There was another med I was taking a long time ago called Lytho. That one was good but it made me gain a lot of weight. I was at 280 pounds. Those pills would have me too relaxed. I was so out of it I would even drool on myself, especially at nighttime.

JUANITA: What effects do all these pills have on you?

LALIA: Well, I have taken some meds that make me faint. At times I even get diarrhea. Another medication that made me gain a lot of weight was Prozac. But I can't live without Prozac even if they make me gain weight. *Sin las Prozac me vuelvo loca. Me ponen mi mente relax.* [Without my Prozac I would go crazy. They relax my mind.] I know my meds. The doctor wanted to put me on Xanax but I had taken them before and knew they did not work for me. I have tried them all. I know which ones work for me and which ones are not good. I don't know what is wrong with [my doctor]. He is the only doctor that has prescribed me so many medications. Another thing about this doctor is that with all the meds he gives me, he never checks my liver. Last week I went to the doctor at [the hospital] to get my blood checked and also my liver. Other psychiatrists that I have gone to in the past always would send me to get lab work at least every four months. This one never does. I have gone to do it on my own 'cause taking all those meds can affect the body. . . . *Mis medicamentos son parte de mi vida. Sin ellos no puedo funcionar.* [My medications are a part of my life. Without them I cannot function.] That is why they should be doing blood work. The blood levels would indicate to them if the patients are taking their meds. *Eso esta al garete.* [Literally, "That's adrift," meaning, "That's off the wall, crazy."]

A number of the women either did not take their prescribed medications at all or took them only intermittently, because they were afraid that they might become dependent on them, a commonly expressed fear among minority patients.[34] Pia, who had been diagnosed with depression, explained her concern: "I don't like to take them [the medications] on a daily basis. I don't want to be addicted to them so I only take them when I get nervous." Laurita, also diagnosed with depression, explained why she had decided to stop taking her medication: "I am tired of drinking so many medications. I don't want to be addicted to meds."

A few of the women believed that their ability to overcome their mental illness was directly dependent on God. Like many individuals who attribute their mental illness to religious or supernatural phenomena, these women adhered to their medication only intermittently.[35] Pia remarked, "God helps me. I am asking God to help me set my pills aside."

Some of the women did not understand that their mental illness was a chronic condition that required constant monitoring and attention, including the consistent use of medication. They believed, rather, that they could discontinue the medication once they felt better, much as one might stop taking cough syrup once the cough had vanished. Yadra explained to her psychiatrist why she had ceased taking her antidepressant medication:

DOCTOR: Are you taking meds?
YADRA: I did not take them for two weeks.
DOCTOR: Why?
YADRA: Because I felt better.
DOCTOR: That is a big mistake that people make sometimes. They start to feel a bit better and then leave their medications. Then their condition gets worse.

It is possible that Yadra may have misunderstood the medication regimen. Or she may have simply discontinued her medication as the result of a poor collaborative relationship with her mental health provider or her inability to communicate with him in Spanish, two common reasons for the failure of Latino patients to take their prescribed antidepressant medication.[36] Sabrina's refusal to take prescribed medication, for example, was clearly related to her frustration with her providers. Sabrina, a Spanish-speaking thirty-eight-year-old mother of four, had been diagnosed with bipolar disorder. She provided a lengthy description of her unproductive encounter with a physician to one of the study ethnographers and concluded by saying, "The doctors gave me a prescription. When I was walking out of the hospital I tore up the prescription and kept walking."

Physicians' lack of familiarity with the women's culture or ethnic-specific variations in medication response may have also contributed, at least indirectly, to the women's experiences of side effects from their medication. Latinos may experience greater levels of side effects with some of the medications that are prescribed for mental illness, such as tricyclic antidepressants.[37] Ethnic-specific safety or tolerability levels may be lower for newer-generation antidepressants in comparison with older tricyclic antidepressants.[38] Finally, antidepressant metabolism may also be modified by dietary and other environmental factors that the physician may not have considered.[39]

The lack of appropriate treatment or a failure to adhere to medications necessary to control the symptoms of mental illness could lead to serious consequences for the women and for others as well. Hospitalization may become necessary, particularly if the individual is also abusing substances.[40] Individuals who are not receiving appropriate treatment for mental illness are at greater risk of being victimized by others, and may also be more likely to become violent toward others.[41]

Co-occurring Illness

Many of the women struggled to manage serious co-occurring health conditions in addition to their mental illness, such as obesity—which was sometimes one of the side effects of the medications that they used to manage their mental illness—hypertension, gallstones, asthma, arthritis, lupus, fibromyalgia, and cancer. For example, in addition to the multiple prescriptions that she needed to control the symptoms of her depression, Catalina received ongoing physical therapy and wore a brace on one hand and another one on her leg in an effort to alleviate the symptoms of her severe arthritis and increase her mobility.

Sometimes, the women delayed seeking care for their symptoms, fearful that any care would require the expenditure of money that they did not have. Narcisa explained the consequences of one such decision to postpone seeking medical care for a physical ailment:

> My health has not been the best either. I know I am here because of God's grace. Now, *cualquier cosita que yo me sienta yo vuelo para el*

hospital [any little thing I feel, I fly to the hospital]. Five years ago I had this pain when I would urinate. When I finally went to the doctor's, it was cancer of the cervix. After that I was having problems with my uterus. I had a mass growing on top of my uterus.

Shame and embarrassment also played a large part at times in the women's decision to delay care. Yadra had prevailed upon our ethnographer Isa to accompany her to her doctor's appointment and to remain in the examination room with her while her physician conducted a pelvic exam to determine the source of Yadra's vaginal itching and rash. Yadra confided to Isa that she was embarrassed to tell the nurse and the doctor what the problem was. She was also afraid that the symptoms might be a sign "of the worst," meaning cancer; Yadra's gynecologist had previously told her that they had found "cancerous cells" during her most recent examination. Fortunately, the doctor was able to determine that Yadra's vaginal itching and rash had come about because of her frequent douching and her use of a cortisone cream.

Some of the women believed that the care that they received for these other chronic conditions was not of the highest quality. To some extent, they may have been correct; research has found that individuals with mental illness are at high risk of undertreatment of their co-occurring illnesses.[42] Cesara believed that her inadequate care was due to her financial situation, providing an unknowing commentary on the multi-tiered system of care that currently exists for those with private health insurance, those with public health insurance, and those with no insurance: "*Yo soy un pobre. No soy de familia rica.*" (I am poor. I do not come from a rich family.)

Miranda also was subject to the limitations of the current publicly funded medical care system in the United States. Only thirty-four years old at the time she enrolled in the study and already struggling with the symptoms of bipolar disorder, Miranda suffered a series of three strokes. Our ethnographer Juanita found her curled up in a fetal position in her hospital bed. Miranda complained that it was "a horrible place" and said of the food, "*Lo que dan es una plasta*" (What they give is a blob). Juanita's field notes described the conditions that she observed during her visit: "The conditions of the hospital were pretty impressive. There was a strong foul smell of urine all over the facilities. Everything was dark and dingy."

Inadequate care or delays in the provision of appropriate care for co-occurring illnesses may also be attributable to the health care provider's inability to understand the participant's communication attempts. This may be the result of either the provider's inability to speak the same language as the participant, such as Spanish, or the provider's difficulties in understanding the participant's fractured and disorganized speech, a symptom of the mental illness. In either case, providers may be unable to understand the patient's complaints or, alternatively, may assume because of the communication difficulties that problems simply do not exist.[43]

8

Negotiating Risk

I'm out of control sometimes.
—Katia, explaining her behavior to her psychiatrist

HIV/AIDS Knowledge

We have known for some time now the behaviors that can expose an individual to risk of contracting HIV infection: unprotected intercourse with an infected partner, sharing injection equipment with an infected individual, and transmission from mother to child through the labor and delivery process or breastfeeding. Other behaviors may increase the likelihood of these exposures, including the use of drugs or alcohol prior to intercourse and engaging in the trade of sex for money, food, or other commodities.

Although many of the women in this study could not have explained why such behaviors were associated with HIV transmission, they understood, to a large degree, that they were. In comparison with the low levels of HIV knowledge that have been noted in other studies of HIV risk among severely mentally ill individuals, the participants' level of HIV knowledge was relatively high (Table 8.1).[1] Many had had personal experience with HIV/AIDS through their relations with infected family members and friends. For some, these experiences were sufficient to instill a desire to protect themselves from infection. Teodora, for example, confided,

> I have been drunk in the past. I'm not going to lie to you. I had a blackout last time I got drunk. I would never ever fucking try heroin. My dad is sick with AIDS. He is in a nursing home. I never tried nothing but

> weed and alcohol. I don't want to end up like my dad. I was anti-drug so I can't be smoking, especially with lupus. I will die faster. It's hard, everyone at my house smokes all day.

Mila, also, had learned by watching others that substance use could lead to behaviors that could lead to HIV:

> I don't understand why people keep using drugs. Don't they understand that drugs can lead to AIDS. *Son brutos. Es que no entienden.* [They are dumb. Don't they understand.] It's mainly the young people that don't get it. Well, I think that young people turn to drugs to make themselves feel better and to try and escape from reality. . . . It's the same thing with alcoholics. They can't handle their problems and then they lead to the bigger problem of addiction.

Knowledge, however, can be imperfect. Teodora, for example, realized that the use of heroin could lead to AIDS, but did not know or understand that alcohol may also increase the risk of HIV exposure by lowering sexual inhibitions, impairing judgment, or disturbing the practice of using safer sex.[2] Imperfect knowledge is similarly reflected in the responses that Katia provided to Noemi, a member of our research team:

> NOEMI: Let me know if you think these statements are true or false. Birth control pills protect against the AIDS virus.
>
> KATIA: False. I wish.
>
> NOEMI: If a man pulls out right before orgasm, condoms don't need to be used to protect against the AIDS virus.
>
> KATIA: False. Oh hell no. They better have one or they are not entering.
>
> NOEMI: Most people who have the AIDS virus look sick.
>
> KATIA: False. Some of them be looking good. Shit.
>
> NOEMI: Vaseline and other oils should not be used to lubricate condoms.
>
> KATIA: I heard of people using Vaseline, but that's false.
>
> NOEMI: Latex is the best material a condom can be made of for protection against the AIDS virus.
>
> KATIA: I think that is false.
>
> NOEMI: Cleaning injection needles with water is enough to kill the AIDS virus.

KATIA: False.
NOEMI: Most people who carry the AIDS virus feel and look healthy.
KATIA: False.
NOEMI: Hand lotion is not a good lubricant to use with a condom.
KATIA: False.

Katia recognized that although some people used Vaseline to lubricate condoms, they were either uninformed or misinformed about its ill effects on condoms. Katia was unaware, however, that latex condoms are the best protection against HIV during intercourse and that hand lotion should not be used with a condom in order to maintain the effectiveness of the

Table 8.1. HIV knowledge among study participants (n = 35)

Item	No. correct	%
Birth control pills protect against the AIDS virus. (F)	33	94.3
If a man pulls out right before orgasm, condoms don't need to be used to protect against the AIDS virus. (F)	35	100.0
Most people who have the AIDS virus look sick. (F)	32	91.4
Vaseline and other oils should not be used to lubricate condoms. (T)	28	80.0
Latex is the best material a condom can be made of for protection against the AIDS virus. (T)	29	82.9
Cleaning injection needles with water is enough to kill the AIDS virus. (F)	30	85.7
Most people who carry the AIDS virus feel and look healthy. (T)	30	85.7
Hand lotion is not a good lubricant to use with a condom. (T)	33	94.3
A man is not likely to get the AIDS virus from having sex with a man unless he is bisexual. (F)	35	100.0
Condoms cause men physical pain. (F)	35	100.0
If you're seeing a man and he agrees not to have sex with other people, it is not important to use a condom. (F)	35	100.0
Always leave room at the tip of the condom when putting it on. (T)	35	100.0

Table 8.2. Risk behaviors among study participants (N = 53) during past ninety days and over lifetime

	Past ninety days		Lifetime	
Risk criterion	No.	%	No.	%
Had intercourse with multiple sexual partners and any unprotected intercourse	3	5.7	24	45.3
Had unprotected intercourse with partner believed to have injected drugs or to have had sexual relations with multiple partners	10	18.9	31	58.5
Had unprotected intercourse with partner of less than twelve months, and is uncertain whether partner had sexual relations with others or injected drugs	9	17.0	29	54.7
Had unprotected intercourse with partner known to be HIV-positive	0	0.0	5	9.4
Had unprotected intercourse with partner of unknown HIV serostatus	12	22.6	28	54.9
Shared injection equipment	1	1.9	4	7.5
Total number of individuals reporting at least one high-risk behavior	14	26.4	36	67.9

condom. Although it seemed initially that she understood that individuals with the AIDS virus may not look sick, she failed to recognize that the majority of individuals who are infected may look and feel healthy. Nevertheless, she understood, at least intellectually, the risk that was associated with sexual relations with multiple partners. She explained to our ethnographer Isa what she would do if her partner was engaging in sex outside of their relationship:

KATIA: I trust myself with condoms 'cause I'm worried about AIDS. Even smart people get AIDS. You don't put on a condom, then no foreplay then. I even buy them. I get embarrassed. I got tested not too long ago. I don't believe it, it was an anonymous test. People should not get embarrassed talking about cleaning their needles. Shit, if you use them, stay safe. I would not get embarrassed cleaning my needles.

ISA: What would you do if you found out your man was sleeping around, Katia?

KATIA: Shit! Kick his ass if he is sleeping with another woman.

ISA: You said you had a HIV test, right? How did it feel waiting for the results?

KATIA: I was nervous the whole time.

We had been concerned even before we began recruiting for the study that many of the women might not understand how HIV is transmitted and how they could protect themselves from contracting the infection. Ethically, we could not, we believed, observe the women over a period of time as they repeatedly exposed themselves to risky situations. Yet we could not intervene in each such instance because, by doing so, we would be changing the very context that we were trying to understand in order to develop a targeted, systematic intervention that could be implemented and tested.

In order to address this ethical issue, we had provided each study participant at the time of her enrollment with basic information about HIV transmission and prevention and a listing of community resources where she might obtain HIV testing and counseling, substance use treatment, and assistance with issues related to family violence. It became clear to us, as evidenced by Katia's responses above, that this information was only partially digested.

Even if the women had been able to absorb all of the information that had been provided to them, knowledge is generally insufficient to bring about a change in behavior.[3] Despite the variation that exists across the numerous theoretical models that are utilized as the basis for HIV risk reduction interventions, there is general agreement that, in addition to receiving information, individuals must be able to relate the information to their own situations in order to recognize risk, must have sufficient motivation to modify their behavior, and must develop the behavioral skills necessary to do so.[4]

Perceiving Risk

Within the general population, individuals often tend to underestimate their risk of contracting HIV, frequently because they assume that others think and act as they do. Individuals with a severe mental illness may have even greater difficulty perceiving and assessing their HIV risk accurately.[5] Absent the application of their knowledge to their own situations and actions, so that there is a recognition and understanding of the connection between their own behavior and their disease risk, individuals may have little incentive to change their behavior.[6] Such was the case with the majority of the women who participated in this study; although many were at extremely high risk of contracting HIV/AIDS, either because of their own sexual and drug-related behaviors or because of their partners' actions, they did not perceive that they were, indeed, at risk (Table 8.2).

Katia, for example, seemed completely unaware of the relationship between having unprotected sexual relations with multiple partners and HIV risk. She described a sexual relationship she had previously had with a married man. Her concerns at the time focused only on the unanticipated pregnancy that had resulted. Katia placed great faith in her current partner's representations that he was not involved sexually with anyone other than Katia:

> Back in New Jersey I dated a married man for three years . . . five years ago. Since he was married I promised him I will never interfere with his family. I became pregnant and told him. He told me I would have to get an abortion. At the time I was smoking crack but he never found out about this. He had heard rumors at the bar that I

> was smoking crack. He confronted me but I denied it. I loved him but he was never going to be mine, when I left I told him this is it. He told me he was going to go back and work things out with his marriage. I don't have to worry about that with [my current partner] because he is mature and I am the only person he is sleeping with. [My current partner] doesn't use a condom and he doesn't like them so he won't use them.

Many of the women in our study who had steady partners believed that their partners, like themselves, were monogamous. Accordingly, they assumed that safer sex precautions, such as condoms, were unnecessary and did not discuss the issue with their partner. This is not surprising because, in general, individuals involved in intimate relationships tend to view their partner in the best possible light, and may even ignore or distort details that are inconsistent with that perspective.[7] They often see their intimate partner like they see themselves and consequently believe that their partner is a good person.[8] This process, known as the false consensus effect, may lead individuals to perceive inaccurately their intimate partner's HIV risk behaviors and, consequently, to misjudge the extent to which they are themselves at risk of exposure to HIV as a result of their partner's behaviors.[9]

Yadra was one of the few women in the study who seemed to use her knowledge of HIV transmission and prevention in her own life, taking affirmative steps to reduce the possibility that she might be exposed to the virus. She explained to one of our ethnographers how she went to special lengths to ensure her own protection:

> JUANITA: When you guys have sex do you use protection?
> YADRA: Oh yes. That is the only way. I don't trust anyone.
> JUANITA: Who provides the condoms, him or you?
> YADRA: *Yo los compro por que y si se pone uno que tiene un roto.* [I buy them because what if he puts one on that has a hole.] I don't trust anybody.

Later, however, when we learned that Yadra had contracted chlamydia from her partner, it became clear that she and her partner were not using condoms during their sexual activities, at least not consistently, and that her partner had been having unprotected sexual relations outside of their relationship. After confronting her partner with the fact of her infection, she told us that she had broken off the relationship and sought HIV testing:

> YADRA: I took everything. I left him with shit . . . I did an HIV screening while I was taking the classes at [the vocational training center].
>
> JUANITA: Did you get the results?
>
> YADRA: Yeah, I had to call a phone number. My results were negative, thank God.
>
> JUANITA: That is good. How often do you get tested?
>
> YADRA: Well, I get tested any time I have the opportunity but at least once a year.

There are many factors that may have influenced Yadra to have unprotected sexual relations with her partner, despite her apparent knowledge of the link between HIV transmission and unprotected sex. These are discussed in greater detail in the following section, which deals with risk in context.

Yadra's efforts to ascertain her HIV status are consistent with the long-standing wisdom suggesting that HIV testing constitutes a key component of HIV prevention.[10] According to the 2001 Behavioral Risk Factor Surveillance Study, 46 percent of U.S. adults have ever been tested for HIV.[11] In our study, 62.9 percent of the thirty-five women responding to our questions about HIV testing indicated that they had obtained an HIV test during the preceding year, a proportion falling midway between the 11 percent and 89 percent prevalence for lifetime testing that has been documented in other studies.[12] Consistent with previous research, we found that a greater proportion of our participants with a nonpsychotic disorder, that is, with bipolar disorder or major depression but not schizophrenia, had been tested for HIV.[13]

Some of the women spoke about the risks of HIV that they saw in the behavior of others, but they were unable to apply this understanding to their own situations. Laura, for example, often fretted about the risks that her gay brother faced by having multiple sexual partners: "I tell him one of these days he is going to go through something scary like a illness or something. . . . My brother is addicted to sex. . . . He quickly moves on to another dick. I tell him but he doesn't listen." Despite this insight,

Laura had a succession of sexual partners during the course of the study and rarely, if ever, used condoms.

Risk in Context

It is only by viewing HIV risk in the larger context of the women's lives that it is possible to understand how their various circumstances, even those that were not of their own making, ultimately converged to increase their risk of HIV infection. It is all too easy to point a finger and admonish individuals for their refusal or failure to use condoms during intercourse, for their continued use of drugs, for trading sexual favors for various commodities. However, the majority of the women in this study were born into a constellation of circumstances and events that destined them to difficult lives. Indeed, it is difficult to discuss each circumstance singularly, for each has implications for the others, creating a patchwork of seamless and overlapping traumas in a never-ending drama.[14] One such factor standing alone might be surmountable; multiple factors in concert, without adequate support from critical others and health care providers, make the avoidance of an increase in HIV risk nothing short of remarkable.

Genesis of Risk: Childhood Abuse

Childhood abuse has been linked to an increase in HIV risk through complex pathways. Childhood sexual and physical abuse are associated with mental illness during adulthood,[15] substance use among individuals with and without severe mental illness,[16] and an increased risk of sexual and physical abuse in adulthood.[17] The interaction between trauma and severe mental illness may lead to more severe psychiatric symptoms, an increased risk of relapse, and revictimization[18] and has been associated with unprotected sexual intercourse and substance use.[19] Multiple traumatic episodes may increase the likelihood that symptoms of the mental illness will persist.[20] Childhood sexual abuse, in particular, may lead women to believe that they have little or no control in later relationships and little ability to effectuate change,[21] thereby laying the foundation for participation in high HIV risk behaviors that do not occur until far in the future, such as unprotected sexual relations, trading sex for money or drugs, and engaging in sexual relations with partners who inject drugs.[22]

Three-quarters (75.5 percent) of the women in our study had been the victims of either sexual or physical violence, or both, during their childhood. Many of the women were later victims of partner violence. Some, like Zamara, who had been diagnosed with major depression, came to believe that such abuse was a normal part of every relationship, signifying love:

> Daniel abused me for years. I needed to get away before he killed me. Daniel even broke my ribs. [*Pointing to her hands*] Daniel used to tie me up and hit me. I left because of the situation and entered a bad situation as well. My parents used to hit me as a punishment and still do so I thought hitting was part of the relationship with Daniel. My mom always hit me and loved me at the same time. Daniel was married and had a fifteen-year-old son living with him. Before I left Puerto Rico, Daniel got a girl pregnant. Daniel told me I had to help him take care of the baby. Daniel was an evil man. . . . He liked to fight and hit me and then have sex. He even tried to sexually abuse his own daughter. Daniel said he felt sorry for women because he believed women were put on this earth to suffer.

Many of the women who had been abused as children also used drugs. Although substance use is often used as a coping mechanism by women who were sexually abused as children, we cannot know whether the women initiated their substance use as a way of coping with the emotional pain of their abuse.[23] Nevertheless, the possible connection between the pain of the abuse and dependence on drugs seemed clear to a number of our participants and to their mental health care providers. Isa, one of the ethnographers, recorded the following notes during her attendance with Marisa at a group therapy session, during which an audio recording could not be used:

> [The provider] said that eight to nine out of ten women that visit their offices for counseling have abuse issues of some type that have not been resolved. She said that unresolved issues is the largest cause that leads people to use chemicals to numb the pain. One of the ladies said, "*El ligao, three ligaos y se me adormesia todo.*" [The mixes, three mixes and everything would be numbed.] Another lady said that they blame

everything else on everyone except themselves. She said, "*El perico—te hablo de mi tio, la tia, el primo. Te hablo de todo el mundo, menos de mi.*" [The weed—I will talk about my uncle, my aunt, the cousin. I will talk about everything except about me.]

Cognitive Development and Impairment

Symptoms of the severe mental illness itself may heighten HIV risk. Individuals with schizophrenia, for example, may be unable to evaluate accurately the risk associated with the various situations they encounter because of impairments in those areas of the brain that are responsible for higher-level executive functioning, such as reasoning and problem solving.[24] Attention deficits decrease the likelihood that individuals will recognize environmental cues that may signal danger or risk, while memory impairments reduce the likelihood that previous dangerous encounters and locations will be remembered and avoided.[25] Substance use may result in further impairments in abstract reasoning, learning, and information processing,[26] particularly among women.[27] HIV risk may be further compounded by illness-associated deficits in social skills, such as an inability to form lasting relationships, an inability to negotiate solutions to conflicts, and a lack of assertiveness, characteristics that may increase the likelihood that an individual will acquiesce to risk-laden demands imposed on them by others.[28] As a result, compared to women without a severe mental illness, they may be more likely to have a greater number of sexual partners, to have a greater number of unplanned pregnancies, to exchange sex for money or other commodities, and to be victims of violence.[29]

Individuals with an affective disorder, such as bipolar disorder and major depression, may be at even greater risk of HIV infection. A study of Medicaid claims and welfare recipient files of individuals over a two-year period in Philadelphia found that while individuals with a schizophrenia spectrum disorder were 1.5 times as likely to have HIV infection compared to those without a mental illness, individuals with an affective disorder were 3.8 times as likely to be infected as those without a mental illness.[30] During periods of emotional crisis, individuals with bipolar disorder may engage in increased sexual activity, while those with major depression may be more likely to inject drugs.[31]

Miranda, diagnosed with bipolar disorder, failed to recognize the danger inherent in an association with a particular individual. Her lack of judgment in this instance landed her in jail:

> MIRANDA: I was around walking in December when I took a ride from a friend that I have known for years and that knows my family. That's when we got pulled over and I went to jail. I hated being in there. Everyone was fighting all the time. I was there for Christmas and missed my son's birthday. I was scared of the black people in there.
>
> JUANITA: How long were you in jail?
>
> MIRANDA: Two and a half months.
>
> JUANITA: And why was it that you went to jail?
>
> MIRANDA: Because he had drugs and a gun in the car. He told them that I had nothing to do with it from the beginning but they said it did not matter, that they still had to take me in.

Vyna, also diagnosed with depression, recognized that her illness affected not only her ability to make decisions but also her ability to remember what decisions she had made and actions she had taken. She had written in her diary, "Why do I have to make choices? Why can't I make choices? I forgot what choice I made yesterday."

Adolescents with mental illness are even more vulnerable to HIV. They are more likely to engage in sexual encounters at a younger age and to have a greater number of sexual partners compared to youth who do not have a psychiatric diagnosis.[32] These behaviors may result from the effects of the mental illness on their decision making ability, reality testing, level of impulsivity, and social interaction.[33] As is the case for adolescents in general, other aspects of their social environment, such as the nature of their interaction with their parents, the availability of appropriate adult role models, and peer influences, may interact with individual-level factors to increase (or decrease) HIV risk.[34]

Teodora, for example, seemed to have experienced moods at a young age that are suggestive of the bipolar disorder that now affects her. It is difficult to know whether her early interest in sex was fueled by the impulsivity associated with this diagnosis or by the impulsivity that is a corollary of normal adolescence. Regardless of its source, the consequences of Teodora's multiple sexual liaisons at a relatively early age are now sobering to her:

TEODORA: Just like herpes at the age of fourteen affected me. [*Covers the side of her mouth and lowers her voice*]

ISA: How did herpes affect you?

TEODORA: At fourteen years old I thought I was the shit. I could get any man I wanted and I was really sexually active. I wasn't a whore but I had a lot of sex. After I got herpes I stopped sleeping around.

Getting By in the 'Hood

Like the majority of individuals with severe mental illness, the participants in this study lived in poor, inner-city neighborhoods characterized by ubiquitous violence and high rates of substance use and sexually transmitted infections.[35] The five areas of Cleveland that the majority of our participants called home, and in which they encountered their sexual and drug-sharing partners—Clark-Fulton, Detroit Shoreway, Hough, Ohio City, and Tremont—were also home to the highest numbers of individuals living with HIV/AIDS.[36] Because of this high prevalence of HIV/AIDS, the participants were more likely by chance alone to come into contact with individuals who were HIV-seropositive than if they had lived in an area with a lower prevalence of HIV-infected individuals.

Many of the participants were themselves victims of indiscriminate violence. Delfina had been robbed at gunpoint, leaving her without adequate funds to meet her living expenses: "I was coming home from work and I had money with me. All the money I had made that night. It was around three a.m. They put a gun to my neck and I had to give up all my money." Another participant had been raped, directly exposing her to the threat of HIV. While between 14 and 25 percent of adult women in the general population may be exposed to sexual assault, anywhere from 21 percent to 38 percent of women with a severe mental illness may experience rape as an adult.[37] The ethnographer's notes reflect the conversation, which the participant did not want recorded: "She said she was walking to work down an alley and a guy brutally beat her and raped her. She said that she ended up pregnant from that incident and chose to have an abortion. She said that her own family does not know of the incident because she was too scared to tell them."

Even the young children of our participants were not spared from the violence. The notes of one of our ethnographers recount the rape of Laurita's two young daughters by a trusted family friend. The trauma exacerbated Laurita's depression, plunged her son into a deep depression because he had been unable to protect his sisters from the abuse, and likely set into motion a chain of shorter- and longer-term consequences that potentially include an increased risk of revictimization and HIV for Laurita's daughters in the future:[38]

> Laurita called the office crying and . . . told me she needed help. I asked her what happened. She said that [the family friend] raped her daughters over the weekend and she needed to get them help. He . . . touched Evelyn and tied Cristina's mouth with a bandana she was wearing on her head. Laurita said that he fingered her until the point of making her bleed. When he attempted to take his pants off, Cristina was able to get away. Laurita said that it appears this was not the first time that he had taken advantage of little girls. Her sister-in-law that used to live in that house was also friends with him and it appears that he had also fondled her daughters. She said that the detectives are investigating. Laurita said that she is very overprotective with her kids and the only reason he was around was because he was a family friend and had been trusted for years. He was good friends with her son, and used to come over and play video games with him. Laurita said that her son feels guilty because he was not able to protect his sisters. She said that he has spent his time locked up in his room and refuses to come out and talk. He is saying that he is going to kill [the family friend] for what he has done. Laurita said she does not know when the kids are going to return to school. She said they have all been sleeping with her on her bed because they are scared someone is going to come into their room.

The women's relative lack of resources frequently challenged them to identify creative strategies to pay for needed goods and services. For some, this meant trading sexual favors for food, shelter, drugs, and other necessities, a practice that entails significant risk of HIV and of violence as well.[39] Women, more than men, may be forced to engage in "survival sex" in order to survive their living situations.[40] And because these exchanges occurred within parts of the community characterized by a relatively high prevalence of HIV/AIDS, the women's risk of contracting HIV through such exchanges was even greater than it might have been in another context.[41] Despite her knowledge about HIV transmission, and her threat to "kick ass" if she were to learn that her partner had been having sexual relations outside of their own relationship, Katia often used sexual favors as a form of barter, such as with her mechanic in exchange for the use of a car and car repairs. During one shadowing session, she told the ethnographer, "I need to call my mechanic. The mechanic likes me and he gave me a car. I had him like that [sexually]." She laughed. Then the phone rang; it was the mechanic. "I'm going to see him and then I'm going out to lunch. You see how I got this man." We knew from various other conversations that these "lunches" were condom free.

Sex and Drugs

Substance use has been correlated with a greater level of sexual activity, with having multiple partners, and with sex trading.[42] However, the relationship between substance use and sexual behavior is a complex one and can be influenced by numerous other factors. These include environmental factors, such as poverty and social networks; the individual's level of impulsivity and thrill seeking; social competence; and cognitive expectancies.[43] Alcohol, for example, appears to heighten individuals' risk-taking intentions through subjective sexual arousal, even though there may be no physiological genital arousal, suggesting that other factors may be important as well.[44]

We noted in Chapter 2 that Hermosa had begun to use heroin again, after her then-partner reintroduced her to it. Hermosa's injection drug use put her at risk of HIV directly, as a result of sharing injection equipment.[45] Honoria, however, was at indirect risk of contracting HIV through injection drug use. Honoria did not inject drugs, but her husband, Alfredo, with whom she engaged in unprotected sexual relations, did, and regularly shared equipment with other men who also injected heroin, not knowing, and perhaps not caring, whether they were infected with HIV. Our ethnographer recorded her visual observations during one shadowing episode at Honoria's apartment:

> Alfredo walks in the apartment. He slams the door open and in anger begins to throw things and punches the wall. He goes in the bathroom and begins talking. During the audio recording he walks across the living room and bathroom. The last fifteen minutes of the recording/visit he sits between the living room and the dining room. The

apartment is small so he sat on his knees right next to the exit door. He answers Honoria and his eyes begin to close. His head tilts frontward. His arms are resting next to his torso. His arms are black and blue and swollen. He has old cut marks on his wrists. Sweat came down his eyes and cheeks. He looked at me twice and apologized for me seeing him like that. As I opened the door to leave I told him to watch his fingers because they were slightly under the door. He looks at me and mumbles quietly. Meanwhile, Honoria sits on the sofa and cries.

Because Alfredo shared his injection equipment with others whose HIV status may have been unknown to him, Alfredo may have contracted HIV from a man who was infected with HIV. Absent an HIV test, which he had not obtained, it was impossible to know whether he was infected. And if Alfredo were infected with HIV, there is a high probability that the infection would have been transmitted to Honoria through their frequent unprotected sexual intercourse.

People with mental illness and a co-occurring substance use disorder are more likely to be victimized than individuals with either a substance use or psychiatric disorder alone.[46] It is believed that cognitive deficits and relative social isolation related to mental illness may impair individuals' ability to evaluate accurately the trustworthiness of others and the safety of their circumstances. Additionally, substance use can affect areas of the brain that are responsible for judgment, decision making, and impulse control.[47] Consequently, the individuals may become easy targets for others when they are in search of or under the influence of a substance.[48] Julieta, for example, had been diagnosed with major depression and, although she was not alcohol dependent, she often used alcohol excessively. In a conversation with her sister, Ida, her mother, LaReina, and one of the study ethnographers, she recounted her rape and the events leading up to it during the previous evening:

JULIETA: Well, I went out to the bar and had a couple of drinks. I remember leaving the bar and going to my friends' house. Next thing you know I don't remember anything.

ISA: What bar was this?

JULIETA: [Bar 1]. Well, we went to [Club 2] after [Bar 1]. I don't remember going to [Club 2]. A taxi brought me home at four a.m.

IDA: She got here all beat up and dirty.

ISA: Dirty like how?

IDA: She had dirt all over her face and blood on her face.

ISA: Oh my God. I'm sorry you had to go through that.

IDA: I told her she can't be drinking like that. In a way, it's her fault. She is crazy. I would never do the things she does.

ISA: Did you go the hospital? You don't remember anything whatsoever, Julieta?

IDA: Yeah, I called the ambulance and they took her.

JULIETA: I can't believe that happened to me.

ISA: I'm sorry, are you OK?

JULIETA: Yeah. Thank God all the tests came back fine and I don't have anything. I went out with a group of friends and they said I was messed up.

IDA: Man, what kind of friends are those?

ISA: What do your friends say about what happened? Did they say anything?

IDA: I heard they [the men who raped her] threw her out of the porch into the yard, that's how she got dirt on her face.

JULIETA: They found condom residue so I'm glad a condom was used. Doctors gave me pills to prevent any STDs.

ISA: What time did this all happen?

IDA: She got home at four a.m.

JULIETA: I don't remember anything.

IDA: These people are crazy. But it's Julieta's fault for being raped.

ISA: Why do you say that?

IDA: Because she leaves from the bar with anyone.

JULIETA: I'm doing better now. My friend is a bouncer at [Club 2] and he'll watch out for me. He said from now on he is gonna see. I mean, I'm OK now. I'm not going to let it get to me. We are going out tonight.

Because we do not know all the circumstances that led up to Julieta's rape, and Julieta is unable to recall them, we do not know to what extent her judgment may have been impaired with respect to decisions, if any, that she made as she became increasingly intoxicated. Regardless of what these decisions may have been, it is clear that her intoxication increased her level of vulnerability to danger and exploitation, and the men who raped her used that increased vulnerability for their own ends. And although Julieta's mother and sister were able to see the connection between Julieta's usual behavior at the clubs and her vulnerability to rape,

Julieta either could not or did not want to acknowledge the possibility of an association.

Julieta's rape may, as well, be related to the childhood abuse that she experienced. Early sexual abuse may increase an individual's vulnerability to revictimization in adulthood.[49] Many individuals attempt to cope with the trauma of rape through a variety of ways, some of which may be self-destructive: excessive drinking, self-blame, and sexual risk.[50] Julieta already uses these self-destructive coping strategies; this rape may lead to an exacerbation of her drinking and her sexual risk taking through the indiscriminate selection of sexual partners at the clubs that she frequents, and thus to an even higher level of HIV risk.

Cultural Values, Gender Role, and Risk

The traditional gender norms associated with the cultural scripts of *machismo*, *marianismo*, and *familismo* may operate so as to heighten or diminish HIV risk. The more negative dimensions of machismo, marianismo, and familismo may lead to an increase in HIV risk. *Machista* males may seek to establish their masculinity and virility through sexual encounters with multiple partners, dominance of women, and excessive alcohol use.[51] Some Latino men may believe that "once ignited, [their sexual desire] is beyond their control."[52] Women who adhere to the *marianista* tradition may feel compelled to acquiesce to partner demands, to remain passive in sexual interactions, and to maintain silence with respect to sex and sexuality ("sexual silence").[53] The loyalty to the family demanded by familismo may further reinforce the women's felt obligation to obey her partner.[54] Safer sex may be perceived as immoral, at least in part because its use requires communication related to sexual needs, which contravenes the prescribed gender script for women.[55] The enactment of such scripts may lead to the man's refusal to use condoms and the woman's inability to negotiate safer sex. The most extreme scenarios may include sexual coercion or partner violence, which can lead directly and indirectly to increased HIV risk.[56]

Researchers have noted that even when Latinas accurately perceive that they are at risk of HIV through unprotected sex with a possibly nonmonogamous partner, they may hesitate to protect their own health through the use of condoms during sexual relations.[57] Their efforts to do so may be impeded by gender role scripts that demand both submissiveness in sexual decision making and the sacrifice of personal needs in order to sustain the relationship.[58] A woman's failure to conform to these sexual norms may prompt others in her social milieu to characterize her as a "bad" woman or a "flirt girl" engaging in promiscuous behavior.[59] Such a characterization carries additional implications for both the woman's own self-esteem and, as a consequence, the nature of her future romantic and sexual relationships and interactions. Indeed, a "woman's identity rests not only on her own behaviors but on her partner's actions and others' appraisals and evaluations of her actions."[60] The expectation of submissiveness may have especially significant implications for young Puerto Rican girls, who are more likely to have a significantly older partner at first intercourse, an occurrence that is often sanctioned by the girl's parents in the belief that the older man will be more likely to provide adequate support to the family.[61]

Teodora found herself in such a situation with Brian, who regularly abused her and then demanded—and took—the sex that he wanted, suggesting that what was portrayed as sexual relations was, in fact, the establishment and re-establishment of Brian's dominance and power within the relationship. Teodora remained confused by Brian's motivations and by her own willingness to stay with him under such circumstances: "I'm falling out of love with Brian. Brian is really fucking up my head. He told me he fucked this fifteen-year-old. Right after he hits me. He wants to have sex. It doesn't feel good. 'Cause he just finished hitting me. He doesn't give me a choice, he gets on top of me. . . . I don't know why I'm with him. . . . I don't know if I'm scared of him or being by myself."

It would initially appear that the more positive qualities associated with these same constructs would act to reduce HIV risk and ensure a stable and relatively HIV-risk-free partner interaction. The positive qualities of machismo, such as the protection and support of one's family and the demonstration of respect for women, suggest that the male partner would not engage in sexual liaisons outside his primary intimate relationship.[62] Similarly, marianismo demands that a woman have only one sexual partner, while belief in and enactment of familismo suggests that priority is to be given to the family and its needs. However, it appears that increased support from the male partner that fosters the woman's dependence on the partner may actually increase vulnerability to HIV infection. One study of 187 Puerto Rican women between the ages of eighteen and fifty-five found that the women who relied on their partners for material assistance, such as money and help with child care demands, developed a degree of dependence on the male partner that was associated with decreased condom use.[63]

The ten women in the study who had sexual or romantic relationships with women were also at risk of HIV infection, despite the relatively low risk of woman-to-woman transmission.[64] Like the majority of the participants who had sexual relationships with men only, these women were unable to apply their knowledge to their own situations, believing that their sexual activities were not risky, despite their objective risk,[65] or that, as lesbians, they could not be at risk.[66] Elena, for example, explained to our ethnographer Isa during a shadowing episode, "I'm clean because I only be with women and not men. There's not protection for women lesbians. . . . I don't sleep with men."

Six of the women also maintained sexual relationships with men, leaving them vulnerable to infection by their male partners, none of whom were willing to use condoms. The cultural value of *hembrismo* encourages women to remain submissive to men, even while pursuing their own goals; perhaps the women were able to maintain a safe and acceptable identity within their Latino community by engaging in relations with men while they simultaneously pursued the relationships with women that provided them with emotional and sexual satisfaction. Nevertheless, the cultural proscription against same-sex sexual relations weighed heavily on these women, who often felt conflicted about their romantic and sexual partnerships with women. Teodora expressed her torment, exclaiming, "I'm struggling not be gay, I want to be straight. I have issues with God." Many of these women, like Teodora, assumed a facade of heterosexuality in an attempt to find acceptance within the larger Latino community, despite their mental illness. Lalia explained why she was in a relationship with a man, although she always knew that she was *alegre* (gay):

> I can't be gay here. My family doesn't like it. When I lived in Puerto Rico and got married, I still kept my women lovers. The town always gossiped about me. I did eventually tell my mom and brothers, and they said I was disgusting. . . . They think it is not normal, it is a sin. I am trying to have a good life, trying to be with a man, but I don't like to have sex with him, so I tell him it is the drugs [medications for mental illness] so he will not feel bad.[67]

Most of these ten women, however, did not self-identify as gay or lesbian. Already marginalized because of their ethnicity, their poverty, and their mental illness, self-identification as nonheterosexual would likely have resulted in almost complete ostracism from their communities. Woman-woman sex is marginalized within Latino communities.[68] And because sex with men is highly stigmatizing within lesbian communities, the women likely would have been ostracized from the lesbian community had they "come out" as lesbian.[69] These fears were grounded in objective reality and cannot be dismissed as paranoid. Elena explained why she chose to remain "in the closet" about her own sexual orientation: "Mom doesn't really know. I think Mom knows but she doesn't recognize it. Because of the way I look I'm a soft butch. I'm not a femme. I don't wear skirts and stuff like that. I have a cousin that is a lesbian and they treated her bad. They abandoned her. That's why [my girlfriend] doesn't want anyone to know she likes me."[70]

9

Power, Processes, and Agency

I know there's a God.
—Katia, explaining how she survives

Blame is often camouflaged in the language of responsibility. Individuals are responsible for their own poverty; it results from a lack of motivation and industry. Their ill health results from a refusal to take responsibility for their own unhealthy behaviors: smoking, drinking, drug use, overeating. Infection with a sexually transmitted disease results from their own poor judgment, perhaps associated with drinking or illicit drug use but certainly with their unwillingness to use condoms or their unbridled promiscuity. Homeless individuals have brought about their own fate, preferring to spend their time drinking alcohol or using drugs, or maybe refusing to adhere to the medication regimen prescribed for the symptoms of their mental illness. This inclination to blame the victim is founded on a differentiation between "Us" and "the Other":

> Blaming the victim depends on a very similar process of identification (carried out to be sure, in the most kindly, philanthropic, and intellectual manner) whereby the victim of social problems is identified as strange, different—in other words, a barbarian, a savage. Discovering savages, then, is a component to, and prerequisite to, Blaming the Victim, and the art of Savage Discovery is a core skill that must be acquired by all aspiring Victim Blamers. They must learn how to demonstrate that the poor, the black, the ill, the jobless, the slum tenants, are different and strange. They must learn to conduct or interpret research that shows how "these people" think in different

> forms, act in different patterns, cling to different values, seek different goals, and learn different truths.[1]

Indeed, we have known for some time that

> the generic process of Blaming the Victim is applied to almost every American problem. The miserable health care of the poor is explained away on the grounds that the victim has poor motivation and lacks health information. The problems of slum housing are traced to the characteristics of tenants who are labeled as "Southern rural migrants" not yet "acculturated" to life in the big city. The "multiproblem" poor, it is claimed, suffer the psychological effects of impoverishment, the "culture of poverty," and the deviant value system of the lower classes; consequently, though unwittingly, they cause their own troubles. From such a viewpoint, the obvious fact that poverty is primarily an absence of money is easily overlooked or set aside.[2]

However, life trajectories are rarely within the control of any individual. Rather, they reflect a series of choices and actions, some producing favorable results and others not, that are made and carried out in the context of, and in interaction with, our larger society. Nevertheless, despite numerous indications from a multiplicity of data sources, we continue to ascribe to the illusion that individuals are solely responsible for their own fates. As a society, we have chosen to ignore the structural violence and oppression—poverty, racism, segregation, marginalization—that characterize the environments in which the women in this study live their lives and in which they struggle to survive. These forms of social inequality are "*structural* because they are embedded in the political and economic organization of the social world; they are *violent* because they cause injury to people."[3] These forms of violence are ubiquitous and, as such, have become largely ignored as a focus in our efforts to ameliorate disease and improve health.[4]

Researchers have long debated whether the apparent relationship between poverty and the onset of mental illness reflects the movement of mentally ill people toward low-income communities because of their illness symptoms (the geographic drift hypothesis, a variant of the social selection hypothesis) and their loss of employment resulting from their illness symptoms (the socioeconomic drift hypothesis, a second variant of the social selection hypothesis), or whether an individual's risk of mental illness is heightened as a result of poorer economic conditions (the social causation hypothesis). Increasing evidence suggests that, even in the case of mental illnesses for which there exists a strong biological component, such as schizophrenia, the illness is attributable, at least in part, to the direct and indirect effects of lower socioeconomic status.[5] Indeed, one's socioeconomic status has the potential to affect, directly and indirectly, an individual's mental health. There is a continuous feedback between socio-economic status, environmental-level factors, individual-level responses, and the mental health of the individual.

As an example, consider Teodora's situation. Teodora, diagnosed with bipolar disorder, was a high school graduate. She and her daughter subsisted on the sums she received from social security. She resided in an area of the inner city known for its sex work, drug traffic, and violent crime, all of which she confronted each day as she walked out the door. She used drugs and alcohol, and she had engaged in cutting and multiple suicide attempts. It is likely that the rape she experienced during the time of our study (recounted in Chapter 8) will have a psychological and behavioral impact, although we do not know what that effect will be or how much time will transpire before it manifests.

If we were to assign individual responsibility for these events, if we were to Blame the Victim, as it were, we would see only that Teodora was the cause of her own troubles. If she didn't spend her money on drugs and alcohol, she would not be so poor. If she weren't so poor, she could find more suitable housing in a less dangerous area. Yet, while it may be accurate to suggest that Teodora would have more cash at her disposal if it were not spent on alcohol and drugs, it does not follow that the resulting savings would be sufficient to move her beyond a poverty-level subsistence or to afford housing in a more desirable area of the city. Such a conclusion fails to consider the relevant structural factors that affect Teodora's situation and therefore is both simplistic and naive. It is important to consider, as well, the larger context in which Teodora acts out her life.

Growing evidence suggests that the larger environmental context in which one lives may shape the impact of other stressors on individual mental health.[6] Minority populations reside primarily in inner cities; it has been estimated that 90 percent of Latinos live in urban areas.[7] Not infrequently, urban minority populations are highly segregated in less advantaged sections of these urban areas as a result of historical, political, and economic barriers.[8] Many of these cities often lack the economic resources to address adequately the many challenges that exist in densely populated areas, including relatively higher rates of crime, reduced resources to provide health care, and limited educational and occupational opportunities. The social strain resulting from such conditions may adversely affect individuals' mental health. One study, for example, found that individuals' perception of their neighborhoods with respect to vandalism, litter or trash, vacant housing, teenagers loitering, burglary, drug selling, and robbery predicted depressive symptoms nine months later.[9] Another study found that individuals with chronic mental illness have lower mental health care costs and greater residential stability if they are able to reside in newer and properly maintained buildings with fewer units, suggesting that the physical quality of a neighborhood may have a significant impact on mental health.[10]

Teodora, like almost all of the women in this study, was poor, as judged by federal poverty standards, and lived in an area characterized by poverty, high rates of crime, and ubiquitous violence and drug trafficking. Despite these stressful conditions, the police presence has been decreased in these areas as a result of Cleveland's budget shortfall. Publicly funded mental health services, which Teodora and the other study participants desperately need, have been reduced in Ohio's attempt to address its own budget deficit. Each of these actions represents a form of structural violence, however unintended its ultimate impact on individuals may be. Unlike illnesses such as heart disease and cancer, which have been at the forefront of the U.S. public health agenda, mental illness has received significantly less funding for treatment and research.[11] The salaries and benefits afforded to psychiatrists and other mental health professionals working in the public sector, which serves those who, like Teodora, have the most severe symptoms, is significantly less than they might receive in the private health sector. Not surprisingly, as we saw in Chapter 7, the quality of services received by those treated in the public sector may be less than adequate. As a recent report to the federal government observed, "America's mental health service delivery system is in shambles."[12]

Difficulties accessing adequate services may be even more acute for those individuals who have co-occurring substance use disorders. There have been calls for the integration of mental health and substance use treatment services for at least a decade, and some states have instituted this approach to varying degrees.[13] Nevertheless, clients continue to encounter separate treatment systems, each of which insists that the treatment for the comorbid disorder is unavailable until the client has received treatment for the other disorder.[14] Women, and pregnant women in particular, are especially affected; pregnant women are often excluded from substance use treatment programs, specifically because of their pregnancy, and denied mental health treatment services because of their failure to address their substance use issues.[15] And even if treatment is potentially available, the lack of structural accommodations to support and facilitate treatment, such as child care, parallel treatment for children, and residence of the children with their mother while she is in treatment, may preclude participation in or successful completion of treatment.[16]

Even assuming that Teodora were able to obtain employment in Cleveland's deteriorating economy, it is unlikely that she would have been able to earn much more than she was receiving through social security. One study found that unemployed mentally ill individuals subsisting on disability payments and rental subsidies derived a monthly income that was only slightly less than that received by individuals employed on a part-time basis.[17] The authors concluded that not only are employment incentives needed, but these incentives must be accompanied by higher paying jobs. Several studies have found that employment opportunities designed specifically to accommodate people with mental illness, such as those with flexible or limited hours or more structured environments ("supported employment"), may not lead to a significant gain in income for the individual or to a significant decrease in publicly funded support for that individual.[18]

Teodora is, indeed, responsible for the choices that she has made with regard to alcohol and drug use. She alone can decide whether to change course and reduce or cease her substance use. But however critical that choice may be to Teodora's life course, it is insufficient in itself to effectuate change for either Teodora or others in a similar situation. Poor minority areas, such as the one in which Teodora lives, are often dis-proportionately targeted by advertising from both the alcohol and tobacco industries,[19] and often have alcohol outlet densities higher than that in non-minority areas.[20] Higher levels of individuals' alcohol consumption have been linked to the proximity and availability of alcohol in the community;[21] to residence in poorly built environments characterized by conditions such as deteriorated buildings, window problems, inadequate heat, and interior water leakage;[22] and to the stress of living in areas that are disordered because of drugs, unemployment, abandoned housing, unresponsive police, and crime.[23] Poor neighborhood conditions have also been found to have a negative effect on the likelihood that individuals will complete an alcohol treatment program.[24] Completion of treatment necessarily assumes that such treatment is even available and accessible through publicly funded health care mechanisms or that the self-help program Alcoholics Anonymous is adequate for all those who wish to cease their alcohol use.

Consider, as well, the impact of structural forces on the very composition of and dynamic within the families of these women. Many of them were born into troubled families that were themselves affected by poverty, unemployment, crime, and other forms of institutionalized oppression. The women's abuse as children went unnoticed by a largely dysfunctional bureaucratic system that was charged with the responsibility of protecting children from abuse, but obviously failed to do so.[25] Later, as adults with their own children, they were demonized by the press and politicians for their use of drugs and portrayed as depraved women, lacking any maternal instinct, who would sacrifice the health of their newborns to their drug craze.[26] Many of the women remained in abusive sexual-romantic relationships long after they should have left, believing that they and their children could not be whole in the absence of a father figure, a perspective that was clearly in line with the moralistic exhortations of recent political administrations to preserve the nuclear family regardless of its (dys)functionality.[27]

Individuals who are mentally ill may be politically unable by themselves to effectuate any significant change in this structure. A study published in 2002 found that approximately one-third of the fifty states restricted the rights of people with mental illness to hold political office, to vote, or to serve on juries, representing yet another level of structural violence to those who are labeled as mentally ill.[28] The reasons for their ostracism from the political fabric of society remain undelineated. It is not unlikely, however, that the widespread portrayal by the media of mentally ill people as violent, threatening, and unpredictable has fueled fears of the potential consequences if "these people" were to acquire additional political power.[29]

Efforts to reduce the likelihood of HIV transmission within U.S. subgroups, such as Latinos and individuals who have been diagnosed with a severe mental illness, have focused to a large degree on effectuating change at the level of the individual and, in some cases, their social networks. Some strides have been made in understanding the elements that may be necessary to encourage relatively short-term modification of behaviors that may increase HIV risk among Latinos. Through small and incremental research steps during the almost thirty years of the HIV epidemic, we have learned about the importance of integrating cultural values with risk reduction efforts,[30] the need for a gender-specific focus and setting,[31] the critical role that can be played by peers in the development and reinforcement of collective self-perceptions relevant to HIV risk reduction,[32] and the obvious need to communicate the requisite information and demonstrate the relevant skills in understandable language via a familiar and welcomed modality.[33]

Efforts to reduce HIV risk among individuals with severe mental illness have similarly led to the identification of elements that appear critical to risk reduction, such as exercises that enable participants to understand their own risk of infection and to learn and practice the requisite interpersonal skills to reduce their risk.[34] Despite these gains, one group of researchers concluded in 2003 that the HIV risk reduction interventions that have been developed to date for people with severe mental illness demonstrate "only limited success in helping [them] reduce their HIV risk behavior."[35]

Modifications of existing, evidence-based HIV prevention interventions may be necessary to increase the acceptability and effectiveness of a particular intervention within a specific population.[36] As has been observed previously, HIV prevention interventions for individuals with severe mental illness must be tailored to individuals' diagnostic category, level of functioning, biological sex, and ethnic subgroup.[37] Nevertheless, our efforts to date have failed to heed the numerous and repeated calls for the development of culturally appropriate HIV prevention efforts, as well as culturally appropriate mental health and substance use treatment programs, that are tailored to the social context of the individuals.[38] We continue to homogenize large, diverse groups, seemingly unable to move beyond a reductionist approach to the construction of identity and the corollary compartmentalization of individuals into rigid categories of Latino, person with a severe mental illness, substance user, or woman.

More recent risk reduction and prevention efforts have targeted groups that appear to be at increased risk of HIV because of the high prevalence of risky behaviors within these groups. In doing so, however, researchers have neglected the study of factors within these same populations that may promote resilience and ameliorate or reduce HIV risk. The identification of such factors, particularly those in the environmental domain, could lead to new insights useful to the formulation of more effective risk reduction interventions.[39]

In focusing our efforts on the modification of individual-level behavior to reduce individuals' risk of HIV infection, we have similarly failed to acknowledge and address the structural impediments that stand in the way of long-term behavioral change. The goals and hopes and aspirations of the women portrayed in this volume are no different from those of middle-class white Americans: a safe place to call home, healthy children, a better life. Even as individuals struggle to adopt healthier behaviors, the structural elements that underlie their situations and that may have provided the initial impetus for their unhealthy behaviors continue to exist. Absent the possibility of an important long-term reward, individuals may feel little motivation to forgo the short-term rewards associated with sex or substance use.[40] We must question whether, as researchers, our efforts to empower individuals to make healthier choices are sufficient. Perhaps, in addition, we must sensitize individuals to the existence of alternatives to their current situations and the power of their own agency, as well as advocate for the transformation of the institutional structures that continue to perpetuate poverty, ethnic and gender discrimination and inequality, and the marginalization of those living with mental illness and substance dependence.[41]

Notes

CHAPTER 1

1. Becker, 1963; Lemert, 1951.
2. Poverty was romanticized and street youth heroized by the prolific writer Horatio Alger Jr. (1832–1899). The youths portrayed in his novels lived in urban centers such as New York and Philadelphia. They struggled successfully against adversity and ultimately gained fame and great wealth, the classic "rags to riches" story.
3. Ryan, 1976.
4. Loue, Cooper, and Fiedler, 2003a, b; Loue et al., 2004.
5. Kessler et al., 1994.
6. Cournos et al., 1991; Cournos et al., 1994; Empfield et al., 1993; Meyer, Cournos, et al., 1993; Meyer, McKinnon, et al., 1993; Sacks et al., 1992; Schwartz-Watts, Montgomery, and Morgan, 1995; Silberstein et al., 1994; Stewart, Zuckerman, and Ingle, 1994; Susser, Valencia, and Conover, 1993; Volavka et al., 1991.
7. McQuillan et al., 1997; Steele, 1994.
8. Cournos and McKinnon, 1997, p. 267.
9. Carey, Carey, and Kalichman, 1997; Carey, Carey, Weinhardt, and Gordon, 1997a.
10. Hanson et al., 1992; Kelly et al., 1992.
11. Laumann et al., 1994.
12. Knox et al., 1994; Steiner, Lussier, and Rosenblatt, 1992.
13. Kalichman et al., 1994; McKinnon et al., 1996.
14. Carey, Carey, Weinhardt, and Gordon, 1997a.
15. Aruffo et al., 1990; Carey, Carey, Weinhardt, and Gordon, 1997a; Kelly et al., 1992; Kelly et al., 1995; Knox et al., 1994; McKinnon et al., 1996; McDermott et al., 1994; Otto-Salaj et al., 1998; Sacks et al., 1992; Steiner, Lussier, and Rosenblatt, 1992; Katz, Watts, and Santman, 1994.
16. Katz, Watts, and Santman, 1994.
17. Gearon and Bellack, 1999.
18. Hatters-Friedman and Loue, 2007.
19. Weinhardt, Carey, and Carey, 1998.
20. Brabin, 2001; Hladik and Hope, 2009; Nicolosi et al., 1994; Padian et al., 1997.
21. Centers for Disease Control and Prevention, 2008.
22. Centers for Disease Control and Prevention, 2009.
23. Centers for Disease Control and Prevention, 2006.
24. Anderson and Smith, 2005.
25. Centers for Disease Control and Prevention, 2006.
26. Cleveland Department of Public Health, 2006, 2007, 2008.
27. The samples were drawn to be consistent with counties used for planning purposes by the Ryan White Comprehensive AIDS Resources Emergency Act (C.A.R.E.), Pub. L. 101-381, 104 Stat. 576, which was passed by Congress on August 18, 1990. The legislation established a federally funded program

intended to provide medical care for low income, uninsured, and underinsured HIV-infected individuals and a variety of health-care-related services for them and their families. It is considered to be a payer of last resort. The legislation was named in honor of a child with hemophilia who contracted HIV in 1984 as the result of a transfusion with HIV-contaminated blood. He was expelled from his school after it was learned that he was infected with HIV. Until his death in 1990, he advocated for AIDS research and awareness. Minorities often face multiple barriers in their attempts to obtain services through HIV/AIDS programs. For a complete discussion of these issues, see U.S. Government Accountability Office, 2009.

28. Information pertaining to the purpose and scope of certificates of confidentiality and the application procedure can be obtained through the website of the National Institutes of Health at *grants/noh.gov/grants/policy/coc/*.
29. Sobell et al., 1987.
30. Morrissey and Dennis, 1990.
31. Hough et al., 1996.
32. Twitchell et al., 1992.
33. Sajatovic and Ramirez, 2001.
34. Marín and Gamba, 1996.
35. Miller, Guarnaccia, and Fasina, 2002.
36. Loue, Cooper, and Fiedler, 2003a, b.
37. Loue and Sajatovic, 2006.
38. Loue and Sajatovic, 2006.
39. Onwuegbuzie and Teddlie, 2003.
40. Tashakkori and Teddlie, 1998.
41. Onwuegbuzie and Teddlie, 2003.

CHAPTER 2

1. Good, 1977, pp. 39–40.
2. Guarnaccia, Lewis-Fernández, and Rivera Marano, 2003, p. 353.
3. Low, 1981.
4. Guarnaccia, Rubio-Stipec, and Canino, 1989; Guarnaccia, Lewis-Fernández, and Rivera Marano, 2003.
5. Jenkins, 1988.
6. Guarnaccia, Lewis-Fernández, and Rivera Marano, 2003.
7. Fernández-Marina, 1961; Mehlman, 1961.
8. Guarnaccia, Rubio-Stipec, and Canino, 1989.
9. Gherovici, 2003, p. 138.
10. Lewis-Fernández, 1996; Guarnaccia and Rogler, 1999.
11. Guarnaccia, Lewis-Fernández, and Rivera Marano, 2003; Guarnaccia et al., 1993; Guarnaccia, Rubio-Stipec, and Canino, 1989; Salmán et al., 1998.
12. De La Cancela, 1986; Guarnaccia, Rubio-Stipec, and Canino, 1989.
13. Kleinman, 1996, p. 20. The current version of the *Diagnostic and Statistical Manual* defines "culture-bound syndromes" as "recurrent, locally-specific patterns of aberrant behavior and troubling experience that may or may not be linked to a particular DSM-IV diagnostic category" (American Psychiatric Association, 2000, p. 898).
14. Gherovici, 2003.
15. Downar and Kapur, 2008; Glatt, 2008. While acknowledging the potential role of stress in the development of mental illness, the U.S. public has, in general, distinguished between various disorders in its attribution of causation. A chemical imbalance of the brain has been endorsed as a significant cause of schizophrenia and major depression. Alcoholism has been attributed to factors in the childhood environment, while cocaine dependence is seen as the consequence of a character defect (Link et al., 1999).
16. Bauer and McBride, 2003; Bellack et al., 1997; Torrey and Knable, 2002; Maj et al., 2002; Seeman and Cohen, 1998.
17. E.g., Alvidrez, 1999.
18. Ellman and Cannon, 2008; Castle and Morgan, 2008.
19. Edwards et al., 2003; Gladstone et al., 2004; Levitan et al., 2003; Mulder et al., 1998; Read et al., 2003; Springer et al., 2007.
20. Pribor and Dinwiddie, 1992. It has been estimated that one out of every twenty female clients of a mental health service has suffered childhood sexual

abuse perpetrated by a father (or father figure), uncle, grandfather, or brother/stepbrother (Geanellos, 2003; Kinzl and Biebl, 1991).

21. Morrison, 2001.
22. Allen, Coyne, and Console, 1997; Kilcommons and Morrison, 2005; Kisiel and Lyons, 2001.
23. Briere and Elliott, 2003.
24. Teodora's reference to a "Lifetime movie" reflects the similarity that she perceives between the trauma of her own life and its wished-for fairy-tale ending and that experienced by characters in the dramas that are frequently televised on the Lifetime channel. As an example, the channel recently aired a movie featuring Fantasia Barrino, which was advertised as "the story of a teen mom who overcame a painful past and won *American Idol*."
25. "O" is a street name for the prescription painkiller OxyContin, also known as OC, OX, Oxy, Oxycotton, Hillbilly heroin, and kicker. The drug is used clinically to treat pain associated with fractures, dislocations, back injuries, arthritis, bursitis, and neuralgia. Short-term effects of the drug include feelings of relaxation and euphoria, depressed respiration, constipation, pain relief, and cough suppression. Side effects include nausea, vomiting, constipation, dizziness, sweating, dry mouth, headache, and weakness. Long-term use may result in physical dependence and addiction (U.S. Drug Enforcement Administration, 2010). "X" refers to ecstasy, a popular name for the drug MDMA (3,4 methylenedioxymethamphetamine). This synthetic, psychoactive drug, which is chemically similar to the stimulant methamphetamine and the hallucinogen mescaline, produces feelings of euphoria, emotional warmth, and distortions of tactile experience and time perception. The effects of MDMA include confusion, depression, drug craving, severe anxiety, sleep disturbances, and difficulty with some cognitive and memory tasks. Other effects include muscle tension, teeth gnashing, nausea, blurred vision, chills, sweating, and faintness. Symptoms of withdrawal include fatigue, loss of appetite, depressed mood, and difficulty concentrating. High doses may result in liver, kidney, or heart failure (National Institute on Drug Abuse, 2008).
26. Delgado, 1977; Devereux, 1958; Koss, 1993.
27. The work of the espiritista has been likened to that of a social worker: "Therapists have much to learn from the practices of spiritualists. . . . They know how to work with the extended family and call upon the support of the spiritual community, which militates against that sense of aloneness and alienation so typical to mental illness. Also, there is no stigma as the cause is externalized to spirits. They utilize suggestion, persuasion, and manipulation techniques which Lincoln Hospital psychiatrists in the South Bronx in New York City, one of the largest and most depressed Puerto Rican ghettos, are becoming skilled in applying" (Mizio, 1977, p. 471). And although both psychoanalysis and the advice of an espiritista may involve hypnotic strategies and education in the process of treating a case of nervios, it has been argued that consultation with an espiritista, unlike treatment with a psychoanalyst, ultimately fosters a dependent relationship (Gherovici, 2003). The validity of this distinction is subject to question.
28. Favazza and Conterio, 1988. This compares with estimates ranging from 14 to 750 per 100,000 people in the general population.
29. For research relating to the association between cutting and sexual conflict and risk, see Brown et al., 2005; Suyemoto and MacDonald, 1995.
30. Cuffel, 1996; Regier et al., 1990.
31. National Drug Intelligence Center, 2004.
32. Dixon, Haas, et al., 1991; Khantzian, 1997; Knudsen and Vilmar, 1984.
33. Dixon, Haas, et al., 1991.

34. Gandhi et al., 2003.
35. Koob and Le Moal, 1997.
36. Bifulco and Moran, 1998; Gladstone et al., 2004.
37. Stevens Arroyo, 2000; Wagenheim and Jiménez de Wagenheim, 1994.
38. Lindgren and Coursey, 1995; Phillips, Lakin, and Pargament, 2002; Kroll and Sheehan, 1989; Fitchett, Burton, and Sivan, 1997.
39. Lindgren and Coursey, 1995; Sullivan, 1998.
40. Hansen, 2004a, b; Stevens-Arroyo, 2000; Wagenheim and Jiménez de Wagenheim, 1994; Zea, Mason, and Murguia, 2000.
41. Loue and Sajatovic, 2006, p. 1175.
42. Thaut, 1990; Harper and Bruce-Sanford, 1989.
43. Bunt, 1988.
44. Gold et al., 2005; Hayashi et al., 2002; Talwar et al., 2006; Tang, Yao, and Zheng, 1994.
45. Padilla, 1989, 1990.

CHAPTER 3

1. Lehman, 1995; Ridgeway and Rapp, 1998.
2. Rinaldi and Perkins, 2007; Rothaus et al., 1964.
3. Hall, Smith, and Shimkunas, 1966; Lorei, 1967; Buell and Anthony, 1973.
4. Stevens-Arroyo and Diaz-Stevens, 1982.
5. Rodriguez, 1994.
6. Whalen, 2005.
7. Sánchez Korrol, 1983.
8. Whalen, 2005, p. 8.
9. Baker, 2002; Cruz, 1998; Torres and Velazquez, 1998.
10. Bourgois, 1995.
11. Whalen, 2005; Rivera, 2005.
12. Chenault, 1970; Handlin, 1959.
13. Lapp, 1986; Maldonado, 1979; Piore, 1979; Mills, Senior, and Goldsen, 1950; Perloff, 1950; Richards, 1983; Senior and Watkins, 1966.
14. Campos and Bonilla, 1976.
15. Whalen, 2005.
16. Santana Cooney and Colon, 1996.
17. Bean and Tienda, 1988.
18. Fitzpatrick, 1987.
19. Center on Budget and Policy Priorities, 1988.
20. Borjas, 1985.
21. Rodriguez, 1994.
22. U.S. Census Bureau, 2005.
23. Rodriguez, 1994.
24. U.S. Commission on Civil Rights, 1976.
25. Brookings Institution, 2003; Ohio State University, 1991; U.S. Department of Housing and Urban Development, 2005.
26. U.S. Census Bureau, 2008a, b.
27. Baker, 2002.
28. McKenzie, 2002.
29. Rivera, 2005.
30. Cunningham, Wolbert, and Brockmeier, 2000.
31. Lehman et al., 2002; Marwaha and Johnson, 2004, Rinaldi and Perkins, 2007.
32. Rinaldi and Perkins, 2007.
33. The Personal Responsibility and Work Opportunity Reconciliation Act of 1996, Public Law 104-193, was signed into law by then-president Bill Clinton. This law dismantled the previously existing cash assistance program known as Aid to Families with Dependent Children (AFDC) and replaced it with Temporary Assistance to Needy Families (TANF). The law, which was ostensibly designed to promote family values and encourage self-sufficiency, refashioned the welfare system into a temporary program that would encourage welfare recipients to move from dependency to workforce participation. The legislation established a five-year lifetime limit on the receipt of cash benefits and imposed strict work requirements. In addition, various groups of individuals became categorically ineligible to receive benefits, including many legal immigrants and convicted felons.
34. Bond et al., 2001.
35. Caron et al., 1998.
36. Link et al., 1989.
37. Marchevsky and Theoharis, 2006.
38. WIC is a special supplemental nutrition

program serving low-income pregnant, postpartum, and breastfeeding women, and infants and children up to age five who are at nutritional risk. The federal grant program is authorized by Congress on an annual basis and is available in all fifty states, thirty-four Indian Tribal Organizations, American Samoa, the District of Columbia, Guam, the Northern Marianas, Puerto Rico, and the U.S. Virgin Islands (U.S. Department of Agriculture, 2006). Nutritional risk includes anemia, a history of pregnancy complications, being underweight or overweight, poor pregnancy outcomes, and dietary risks. In general, program participants receive either checks or vouchers on a monthly basis for the purchase of specific food items, such as iron-fortified infant formula, eggs, milk, and cheese.

39. Perese, 2003.
40. In some circumstances, the medication regimen for the treatment of a mental illness must be adjusted or discontinued for pregnancy (Seeman and Cohen, 1998).
41. Link, 1982, 1987; Scheff, 1966.
42. Link, 1987, p. 97.
43. Link, Mirotznik, and Cullen, 1991.
44. Schur, 1971; Becker, 1963.
45. Cook, 2005; Fraser and Shrey, 1986; Muntaner et al., 1993; Marcotte, Wilcox-Gök, and Redmon, 2000; Wilson, 1987.
46. Rosenfield, 1989; Warner and Polak, 1995.
47. McGurk and Mueser, 2004.
48. Platt, 1995; Becker et al., 1998.
49. Rosen et al., 2006.
50. "Section 8" refers to a rental voucher program administered by a public housing authority (PHA) for the benefit of low-income families. In general, the PHA will pay the landlord the difference between 30 percent of the family's household income and the amount determined by the PHA to be the standard rent, which is generally between 80 percent and 100 percent of the fair market rent (U.S. Department of Housing and Urban Development, 2004).
51. Simmons and Singer, 2006.
52. Farmer, 2004; Farmer et al., 2006; Galtung, 1969.

CHAPTER 4

1. Maslow, 1970.
2. The *telenovela*, which can be thought of as a culture-specific form of soap opera, has been referred to as "the most popular type of episodic programming throughout Latin America" (Barrera and Bielby, 2004, p. 4; see also Rogers and Antola, 1985). The *telenovela* not only tells its viewers a story but also provides them with a connection to familiar traditions and their native language. This may be particularly important to individuals on the U.S. mainland, who are separated from their families and friends (Barrera and Bielby, 2004).
3. E.g., Lukianowicz, 1972; Maisch, 1972; Medlicott, 1967; Riszt, 1979. The validity of these findings is uncertain in view of significant methodological problems associated with the conduct of the studies. Many of the studies suffered from selection bias as a result of their inclusion of only women drawn from clinical and forensic samples. Societal standards for female sexual behavior existing at the time the studies were conducted were significantly harsher than they might be today. Additionally, the term "promiscuous," used by some authors to describe resulting behavior, serves only to cast moral judgment rather than to describe in a meaningful way the specific outcome, so that it is unclear what type or frequency of behavior is actually encompassed within that term.
4. Arriola et al., 2005.
5. Loue and Mendez, 2006.
6. Miller, Clark, and Moore, 1997.
7. Hatters-Friedman and Loue, 2007.
8. Goodman, Dutton, and Harris, 1995; Gearon and Bellack, 1999.
9. "To be cured" here signifies wanting

another hit of the drug in order to be cured of the symptoms of withdrawal.

10. Cunradi, Caetano, and Schafer, 2002.
11. Lown and Vega, 2001; Neff, Holamon, and Schluter, 1995; Bushman and Cooper, 1990.
12. Romero-Daza, Weeks, and Singer, 2003, p. 235.
13. Caron et al., 1998.
14. Mattson and Rodriguez, 1999.
15. McFarlane, Wiist, and Watson, 1998a; McFarlane and Parker, 1995.
16. Lower socioeconomic status, language differences, limited access to violence intervention services in one's neighborhood, and lack of transportation may converge to limit women's ability to obtain assistance for partner violence or leave their abusive situations (McFarlane et al., 1997; McFarlane, Wiist, and Watson, 1998b).
17. Dutton and Painter, 1981, 1993.
18. Martinez and Dukes, 1991.
19. Díaz-Olavarrieta et al., 2002; Kantor, Jasinski, and Aldarondo, 1994; Perilla, Bakeman, and Norris, 1994.
20. Vasquez, 1998, pp. 323–24.
21. Scripts serve as cognitive structures that help the participants in an interaction to define the situation, organize the interpretation of events and actions, and guide their performances in the specific episodes (Gagnon and Simon, 1973; Ginsburg, 1988; Metts and Spitzberg, 1996). Through the script, individuals are able to negotiate modifications of their performances and clarify meaning (Metts and Spitzberg, 1996). Communication is critical to the enactment of sexual scripts, which are believed to be determinative of behavioral outcomes at the cultural, interpersonal, and intrapsychic levels (Gagnon and Simon, 1973). At the cultural level, they reflect existing norms that guide the individual in his or her sexual conduct (Gagnon and Simon, 1973). Participants in an interpersonal script use familiar cultural symbols in order to engage with each other. Intrapsychic scripts relate to an individual's sexual desires and preferences and constitute an element in sexual arousal (Metts and Spitzberg, 1996). Research findings suggest that some cultures may endorse partner violence to a greater degree than others through the scripts that have been developed for male and female behavior (Vandello and Cohen, 2003).
22. Galanti, 2003. The negative traits associated with the stereotypical portrayal of machismo reflect to a great degree the pathological view of the psychodynamic perspective. In essence, this perspective conceives of machismo as a hypermasculine response (Panitz et al., 1983) that serves as a defense mechanism (Abad and Suarez, 1975; Diaz-Guerrero, 1955) used in an attempt to overcome dependency, feelings of powerlessness, low self-esteem, or inferiority (McCord and McCord, 1960). These feelings are hypothesized to be the result of being raised as a male in a lower socioeconomic environment, in a matriarchal family, or with a strained father-son relationship. According to this view, males in such situations have a limited array of options through which they are able to exercise power and control and, consequently, adopt a machista orientation (Giraldo, 1972; Patron, 1969). There is considerable debate with respect to both the validity and the importance of machismo within diverse Latino cultures. For these various perspectives as they relate to Mexican culture, see Baca-Zinn, 1982; Benavides, 1992; Cromwell and Ruiz, 1979; Gonzalez, 1982; Mirandé, 1988; Peñalosa, 1968.
23. Galanti, 2003.
24. Loue, Cooper, and Fiedler, 2003b; Pérez-Jiménez et al., 2007.
25. Noland, 2006; Santana et al., 2006.
26. Casas et al., 1994.
27. Bernal and Alvarez, 1983; Mattson and Rodriguez, 1999; Perilla, 1999.
28. Ortega-Vélez, 1998.
29. Sabogal et al., 1987.
30. Alvidrez, 1999.

31. Torres, 1991; Perilla, 1999.
32. Aldarondo, Kantor, and Jasinski, 2002; Kantor, Jasinski, and Aldarondo, 1994; Loue, 2001.
33. Soto and Shaver, 1982; Torres-Matrullo, 1982.
34. Kantor, Jasinski, Aldarondo, 1994; Aldarondo, Kantor, and Jasinski, 2002. West (1998, p. 193), however, has cautioned that "ethnic minorities are not inherently more violent than Anglo Americans; rather, they are more likely than Anglos to be over-represented in demographic categories that are at greater risk for physical violence." Immigration status, country of origin, language, acculturation, and socioeconomic status of immigrants are important considerations in interpreting research findings.

CHAPTER 5

1. Stein, Leslie, and Nyamathi, 2002; Briere, 2002; Wenninger and Ehlers, 1998.
2. Cloitre et al., 1996; Goodman et al., 2001; Meade et al., 2009. There are numerous theories that attempt to explain how childhood abuse may lead to problems in adulthood. For a survey of these various theories, see Hulme, 2004. The relationship between childhood abuse and HIV risk is explored in Chapter 8.
3. Cooley, 1902; Mead, 1934.
4. Cooley, 1902; Demo, Small, and Savin-Williams, 1987; Ross and Broh, 2000; Schwalbe and Staples, 1991.
5. Kruglanski and Webster, 1996.
6. Stangor and Ruble, 1989.
7. Briere and Elliott, 2003; Cloitre et al., 1996; Chartier, Walker, and Naimark, 2007; Edwards et al., 2003; Finkelhor et al., 1990; Muenzenmaier et al., 1993; Mueser, Goodman, et al., 1998; Rosenberg et al., 2007.
8. Finkelhor and Browne, 1985.
9. Wolfe, 1999.
10. Lechner et al., 1993; McCauley et al., 1997; McCrae, Chapman, and Christ, 2006; Springs and Friedrich, 1992; Stein, Leslie, and Nyamathi, 2002.
11. Orellana, 1989.
12. Oberg, 1954, p. 1. The term "culture shock" was introduced by Kalvero Oberg in 1954 to refer to an "abrupt loss of the familiar" or the "shock of the new." Culture shock occurs in various stages or phases, which have been variously termed incubation, crisis, recovery and full recovery (Oberg, 1954, 1960); elation, depression, recovery, and acculturation (Richardson, 1974); and contact, disintegration, reintegration, autonomy, and independence (Adler, 1975). The first stage of elation is characterized by feelings of excitement, which may last for hours, days, weeks, or months. These feelings gradually dissipate, as the individual becomes increasingly aware of the differences that exist between her previous and current environments. This second phase of disintegration is marked by practical problems, an increase in misunderstandings and associated feelings of frustration, a sense of loneliness and uneasiness, and a decrease in self-confidence. During the third stage of culture shock, the individual will begin to reintegrate into the new environment or reject her new situation, blaming others and adopting negative coping mechanisms, such as substance use and self-isolation. During the final stage of recovery, the individual may gradually adjust and adapt to the new environment, experiencing a greater sense of control, autonomy, and belonging (reintegration). Significant variation exists between individuals in their experience of culture shock. The sequence and rate through which they pass through the various stages may differ as a function of their mental state, personality, familiarity with language, family and social support system, religious beliefs, level of education, socioeconomic condition, sex and gender, and past experiences with travel.
13. El-Bassel et al., 2001; Levendosky and

Graham-Bermann, 2001; Muehlenhard et al., 1998.

14. Link et al., 1987; Riskind and Wahl, 1992; Schulze and Angermeyer, 2003.
15. Brockington et al., 1993; Rüsch, Angermeyer, and Corrigan, 2005; Taylor and Dear, 1981.
16. Jones et al., 1984.
17. Angermeyer and Matschinger, 2003; Laing, 1960, 1961; Launer, 1999; Schulze and Angermeyer, 2003. Star concluded from one of the first nationally representative studies focusing on the public perception of mental illness that "mental illness is a very threatening, fearful thing and not an idea to be entertained lightly about anyone. Emotionally, it represents to people a loss of what they consider to be distinctively human qualities of rationality and free will, and there is a kind of horror in dehumanization. As both our data and other studies make clear, mental illness is something that people want to keep as far away from themselves as possible" (Star, 1955, p. 6, quoted in Link et al., 1999, p. 1331). In the case of schizophrenia, it appears that individuals exhibiting positive symptoms, such as hallucinations and delusions, are more likely to be stigmatized and isolated as a result than those who are experiencing negative symptoms, such as a depressed or anxious mood and lack of affect (Lysaker et al., 2007). The extent to which an individual is isolated may vary as a function of the strength of the individual's association with undesirable characteristics.
18. World Health Organization, 2001.
19. Wright, Gronfein, and Owens, 2000.
20. Leaf, Bruce, and Tischler, 1986; Leaf et al., 1987; Rüsch, Angermeyer, and Corrigan, 2005.
21. Link, Mirotznik, and Cullen, 1991; Rüsch, Angermeyer, and Corrigan, 2005; Wahl, 1999.
22. Goffman, 1963; Link, Mirotznik, and Cullen, 1991; Scheff, 1984; Wahl, 1999.
23. Janoff-Bulman, 1992; Walker, 1978.
24. Marshall et al., 2003.
25. The concept of codependency derives from the self-help programs Adult Children of Alcoholics (ACOA) and Al-Anon, twelve-step programs developed to promote recovery for adult children of alcoholics and partners of alcoholics, respectively (Haaken, 1993). Codependency is said to be "characterized by preoccupation and extreme dependence (emotionally, socially, and sometimes physically) on a person or object. Eventually, this dependence on another person becomes a pathological condition that affects the codependent in all other relationships" (Wegsheider-Cruse, 1985, p. 2). Once limited to partners and adult children of alcoholics, the medicalization of caregiving has been extended by some writers to include essentially everyone (Schaef, 1987; Wegsheider-Cruse, 1985). Although the concept of codependency has been popularized through mass media, it is not a diagnosis that is recognized in the *Diagnostic and Statistical Manual, Fourth Edition, Text Revision (DSM-IV-TR)*, the current version of the diagnostic manual published by the American Psychiatric Association that is relied on by mental health professionals for the diagnosis of mental illness. The "diagnosis" of codependency appears to pathologize the caregiving that may be a constituent part of women's moral development (Gilligan, 1982), thereby equating caregiving with pathology. In the context of mental illness, a level of family involvement in the life of the member with severe mental illness may be necessary and even critical to maximize the possibility of recovery, for example, by ensuring adherence to a medication regimen, transporting the individual to medical appointments, and encouraging involvement in social activities.
26. Perese, 1997.
27. Weisman, 2005; Weisman et al., 2005.
28. Capitanio and Herek, 1999; Herek, 1999;

Herek and Capitanio, 1999; McBride, 1998; Reidpath and Chan, 2005.

29. Ritsher and Phelan, 2004.
30. Weisman de Mamani et al., 2007.
31. A significant body of research has been developed that focuses specifically on the burden experienced by caregivers of individuals with severe mental illness. We do not use the term "critical other" synonymously with that of "caregiver," as the latter term implies a more extensive involvement in the provision of various aspects of care than might be expected of a critical other.
32. Clark and Drake, 1994.
33. Horwitz, Reinhard, and Howell-White, 1996.
34. Pinto, 2005; Tolsdorf, 1976.
35. Marín, 1989, p. 414.
36. Bravo, 1989; Salgado de Snyder and Padilla, 1987; Glazer and Moynihan, 1963.
37. Close friends, in addition to blood relatives, may be considered to be part of the family network. *Comadres* and *compadres*, for example, hold a special status in the *compadrazco* system because of historical friendships or because they are the godparents for the children. The network of special relationships is often generational and extends beyond the immediate and extended biological family (Arredondo, Bordes, and Paniagua, 2007).
38. Valenzuela and Dornbusch, 1994, pp.18–19.
39. Triandis et al., 1982.
40. Lugo Steidel and Contreras, 2003. Attitudinal familism has been defined as (1) the feeling on the part of all members that they belong pre-eminently to the family group and that all other people are outsiders; (2) complete integration of individual activities for the achievement of family objectives; (3) the assumption that land, money, and other materials goods are family property, involving the obligation to support individual members and give them assistance when they are in need; (4) the willingness of all members to rally to the support of a member if attacked by outsiders; and (5) concern for the perpetuation of the family as evidenced by helping adult offspring in beginning and continuing an economic activity in line with family expectations and in setting up a new household (Burgess, Locke, and Thomes, 1963, pp. 35–36).
41. Marín and Marín, 1991.
42. Folsom et al., 2005; Caton et al., 1994.
43. Folsom et al., 2005; Koegel et al., 1999; North and Smith, 1993; Padgett, Struening, and Andrews, 1990.
44. Goodman et al., 2001; Kushel et al., 2003; Swanson et al., 2002.

CHAPTER 6

1. Mowbray, Oyserman, and Ross, 1995.
2. Erikson, 1968.
3. Oyserman et al., 2000.
4. Guarnaccia et al., 1992.
5. Galanti, 2003.
6. Kaiser Permanente National Diversity Council, 2001.
7. Ventura, 1994.
8. Bruinius, 2006.
9. Schoen, 2005.
10. Briggs, 1998. An examination of the politics of sterilization reveals interwoven and oftentimes conflicting threads: medical paternalism, Puerto Rican feminist activism, voices of a reproductive rights movement, anticolonialist views, racist undercurrents, and religious conservatism. These themes are inscribed over the very real personal narratives of the women who either chose or were subjected to *La Operación*, as the sterilization procedure came to be called: poverty, unemployment, limited education, high rates of infant mortality, and the unavailability of adequate health care generally and contraceptive information and devices specifically. For an incisive analysis of the political debate, see Briggs, 1998.
11. Schoen, 2005.
12. Schoen, 2005, p. 212.

13. Concerns have been raised about the use of Puerto Ricans as guinea pigs in other experiments as well. Cornelius P. Rhoads, a physician who worked in the Puerto Rico Presbyterian Hospital in the 1930s under the auspices of the Rockefeller Foundation for Medical Research, is alleged to have injected unknowing Puerto Rican patients with cancer cells in order to carry out his cancer research. He is alleged to have claimed, "What the island [Puerto Rico] needs is not public health work, but a tidal wave or something to totally exterminate the population." The U.S. Department of Defense has acknowledged its own role in the conduct of biological and chemical warfare experiments on unknowing Puerto Rican members of the military in 1969. Civilians may have also been exposed (Ruiz-Marrero, 2002).
14. Seeman and Cohen, 1998.
15. Lederman and Sierra, 1994; Ventura, 1994.
16. Belle, 1982; Davenport, Zahn-Waxler, Adland, and Mayfield, 1984; Frankel and Harmon, 1996; Goodman et al., 1994; Hamilton, Jones, and Hammen, 1993; Klehr, Cohler, and Musick, 1983.
17. Rogosh, Mowbray, and Bogat, 1992; Rutter, 1990; Sameroff, Seifer, and Zax, 1982.
18. Levendosky and Graham-Bermann, 2001.
19. Goodwin and Jamison, 1990.
20. Straus, 1991; Straus and Kantor, 1994.
21. Straus, 2001.
22. Straus, 2001, p. 4.
23. Coohey, 2001.
24. Lapalme, Hodgins, and LaRoche, 1977; Nomura et al., 2002.
25. Larsson et al., 2000.
26. Francell, Conn, and Gray, 1988.
27. Lieb et al., 2002; Jaffee and Price, 2007; Kety et al., 1976.

CHAPTER 7

1. Bruce et al., 2002.
2. Harman, Edlund, and Fortney, 2004; Sirey et al., 1999; Wang, Berglund, and Kessler, 2000; Young et al., 2001.
3. Miranda and Cooper, 2004.
4. Alegría et al., 2002; Alegría et al., 2008; Borowsky et al., 2000; Miranda et al., 2002; U.S. Department of Health and Human Services, 2001.
5. Chow, Jaffee, and Snowden, 2003; Young et al., 2005.
6. Sartorius, 2007; Wahl, 1999.
7. Wahl, 1999.
8. Marshall et al., 2003.
9. Wahl, 1999.
10. Collins, 2001.
11. King et al., 2007.
12. Marcos et al., 1973.
13. Marcos, 1976; Rozensky and Gomez, 1983.
14. Marcos and Urcuyo, 1979.
15. Marcos and Urcuyo, 1979. Studies focusing on other illnesses have similarly found that language may pose a significant barrier to health care access and the quality of the care received. In a study of diabetes and hypertension, Spanish-speaking patients whose physicians also spoke Spanish reported higher levels of well-being and functioning than those whose physicians were not fluent in Spanish (Perez-Stable, Nápoles-Springer, and Miramontes, 1997).
16. Disparities also exist in other domains of care. For example, compared to whites and African Americans, Spanish-speaking Latinos are less likely to have a physician visit, an influenza vaccination, or a mammogram (Fiscella et al., 2002).
17. Lopez, 1989.
18. Minsky et al., 2003.
19. Akutsu, Snowden, and Organista, 1996; O'Sullivan and Lasso, 1992; Reeves, 1986; Rogler et al., 1987; Sue et al., 1991.
20. Mathews et al., 2002.
21. Physicians, psychologists, and social workers are to relate to their patients/clients within the ethical bounds established by their professions. In

general, dual relationships with patients/clients, whether business, professional, social, or sexual, are discouraged, whether occurring simultaneously or consecutively; sexual relations with patients/clients are generally prohibited explicitly, even when they appear to be consensual in nature. Some of the ethical standards are enforceable under the provisions of relevant state laws, while others are aspirational. For examples of these ethical codes, see *www.ama-assn.org/ama/pub/physician-resources/medical-ethics/ama-code-medical-ethics/principles-medical-ethics.shtml* (physicians); *www.apa.org/ethics/code2002.html* (psychologists); and *www.socialworkers.org/pubs/code/code.asp* (social workers).

22. Transference, a term that is used in the context of psychoanalysis, has been defined as "a form of displacement involving the redirection of emotions and attitudes from their original instinctual object on to a substitute, especially as occurs in the dependent, child-like, and often sexually and aggressively charged relationship that a person undergoing therapy usually forms with the analyst, generally having features carried over (transferred) from earlier relationships, especially with parents" (Quinn, 2006, pp. 773–74). Transference provides a vehicle by which the individual in therapy can address unresolved aspects of past relationships. In the interactions between Roberta and Mireya, Roberta may not actually have changed at all, but Mireya may believe that she has changed because transference has occurred. Mireya may now attribute to Roberta the characteristics of a loving parent or concerned other.
23. Barrio et al., 2003; Mueser, Bond, et al., 1998; Lawthers et al., 2003.
24. Barrio et al., 2003.
25. Burns et al., 1999; Lamb and Lamb, 1990; Lehman et al., 1999; Quinlivan et al., 1995; Test, 1998.
26. Niquette, Candisky, and Johnson, 2008.
27. Bartels, 2003; Vega and Lopez, 2001.
28. Cramer and Rosenheck, 1998; Rüsch, Angermeyer, and Corrigan, 2005.
29. Schulze and Angermeyer, 2003.
30. As an example, newer antipsychotic medications, known as atypical antipsychotics, are just as effective as the traditional antipsychotic drugs and less likely to cause serious side effects (Daumit et al., 2003; Geddes et al., 2000; Kapur and Remington, 2000; Leucht et al., 1999; Purdon et al., 2000). Atypical antipsychotics include such medications as clozapine, risperidone, olanzapine, and quetapine fumarate.
31. Opolka et al., 2004.
32. Daumit et al., 2003.
33. Foster and Goa, 1999; Kendrick, 1999.
34. Atdjian and Vega, 2005.
35. Alvidrez, 1999.
36. American College of Physicians, 2004; Miranda and Cooper, 2004; Thomson, 2005.
37. Lin, 2001.
38. Plewes et al., 2004; Sánchez-Lacay et al., 2001.
39. Marin and Escobar, 2001.
40. Haywood et al., 1995.
41. Swartz et al., 1998. Individuals with a mental illness are more than twice as likely to be incarcerated as those without a mental illness (Daly, 2006). Approximately 60 percent of jail inmates, 49 percent of state prisoners, and 40 percent of federal prisoners are affected by a mental health problem (Bender, 2006). The increased proportion of inmates with a severe mental illness is due to the convergence of various factors, including the deinstitutionalization of mentally ill people, the relatively limited availability of hospital beds for psychiatric illness, and the relative unavailability of mental health treatment for individuals during periods of incarceration. Many individuals with mental health problems are incarcerated because of violent offenses against others.
42. Lawthers et al., 2003.
43. Bowers, Joyce, and Esmond, 1996; Waxman and Levitt, 2000.

CHAPTER 8

1. Aruffo et al., 1990; Carey, Carey, Weinhardt, and Gordon, 1997a; Hanson et al., 1992; Kelly et al., 1992; Kelly et al., 1995; Knox et al., 1994; McKinnon et al., 1996; McDermott et al., 1994; Otto-Salaj et al., 1998; Sacks et al., 1992; Steiner, Lussier, and Rosenblatt, 1992; Katz, Watts, and Santman, 1994.
2. Dévieux et al., 2007; Robertson and Plant, 1988; Stall, McKusick, and Wiley, 1986.
3. Hanson et al., 1992.
4. The Information-Motivation-Behavioral Skills model posits that the reduction of HIV risk requires adequate information concerning HIV transmission and prevention, the development of motivation to reduce risk, and the acquisition of behavioral skills necessary to do so (Fisher et al., 1994). Various other models have been used as the basis for reduction interventions including, but not limited to, the Health Belief Model (Rosenstock, 1974), the theory of gender and power (Connell, 1987), the transtheoretical model of behavior change theory (Prochaska and DiClemente, 1984, 1992), and the theory of planned behavior (Ajzen, 1991).
5. Carey, Carey, Weinhardt, and Gordon, 1997b.
6. Janz and Becker, 1984.
7. Murray, Holmes, and Griffin, 1996.
8. Higgins, King, and Mavin, 1982; Kenny and Acitelli, 2001; Marks and Miller, 1987.
9. Hammer et al., 1996; Harman, O'Grady, and Wilson, 2009.
10. Centers for Disease Control and Prevention, 2003a.
11. Centers for Disease Control and Prevention, 2003b.
12. Senn and Carey, 2008.
13. Meade and Sikkema, 2005.
14. With respect to the environmental factors, both the type and level of environmental influence are relevant to risk. These factors may occur at the level of interpersonal relations (micro), the level of social and group interactions and institutional and organizational responses (meso), and the level of laws, policies, economic conditions, and other structural factors (macro). The risk environment results from the interplay of inseparable factors operating at multiple levels. Those that have been found to be critical in the social production of HIV risk associated with drug injection include cross-border trade and transport linkages; population movement and mixing, and disadvantaged neighborhoods; the nature of the injecting environment; the impact of peer groups and social networks; the nature of any economic and political transitions; the existence of economic and social inequities associated with sex, gender, and sexuality; social stigma and discrimination; the impact of complex natural and human-made disasters; and the nature and impact of laws and law enforcement policies (Rhodes et al., 2005).
15. Macmillan et al., 2001; Molnar, Buka, and Kessler, 2001.
16. Craine et al., 1988; Goodman et al., 1997; Simpson and Miller, 2002.
17. Arriola et al., 2005; Cloitre et al., 1996; Goodman et al., 2001.
18. Mueser et al., 2002.
19. Malow et al., 2006.
20. Tanskanen et al., 2004.
21. Campbell, 1989; Fellitti, 1991; Hutchings and Dutton, 1993.
22. Klein and Chao, 1995; Miller and Paone, 1998; NIMH Multisite HIV Prevention Trial Group, 2001; Van Dorn et al., 2005.
23. Cunningham et al., 1994; Miller, 1999.
24. Weinberger, 1987.
25. Gearon and Bellack, 1999.
26. Grant, 1987; Grant and Judd, 1976; Reed and Grant, 1990; Verdejo-García et al., 2005.
27. Glenn and Parsons, 1992.
28. Morrison and Bellack, 1987.
29. Miller and Finnerty, 1996.
30. Blank et al., 2002.
31. Sacks and Dermatis, 1994; McDermott et al., 1994.

32. Valois et al., 1997.
33. Brown et al., 1997.
34. Biglan et al., 1990; Fleuridas, Crevy, and Vela, 1997; Rodgers, 1999.
35. Carling, 1995; Wong and Solomon, 2002.
36. Cleveland Department of Public Health, 2009.
37. Koss, 1993; Goodman, Dutton, and Harris, 1995.
38. Goodman et al., 2001.
39. Goodman and Fallot, 1998.
40. Otto-Salaj et al., 1998.
41. Des Jarlais and Semaan, 2009.
42. Weinhardt et al., 2001.
43. Kalichman, Heckman, and Kelly, 1996; Buckley et al., 1994; Fromme, D'Amico, and Katz, 1999.
44. George et al., 2007.
45. Celentano, Latimore, and Mehta, 2008.
46. Sells et al., 2003.
47. Bechara and Damasio, 2002; Finn et al., 1999; Nagoshi, Wilson, and Rodriguez, 1991.
48. Miller, 1999; Miller, Downs, and Gondoli, 1989; Miller, Downs, and Testa, 1993.
49. Arata, 1999.
50. Parillo et al., 2001.
51. Pérez-Jiménez et al., 2007.
52. Marín, 1996, p. 162.
53. Cunningham, 1998; Marín, 2003; Noland, 2006.
54. Ortiz-Torres, Serrano-García, and Torres-Burgos, 2000.
55. Ortiz-Torres, Serrano-García, and Torres-Burgos, 2000, citing Cruz and Serrano-García, 1997.
56. Márin et al., 1997.
57. Dixon, Peters, and Saul, 2003.
58. Amaro, 1988.
59. Faulkner, 2003.
60. Horowitz, 1983, p. 119.
61. Miller, Clark, and Moore, 1997; Driscoll et al., 2001; Márin, 2003.
62. Mikawa et al., 1992.
63. Dixon, Antoni, et al., 2001.
64. Diamant, Lever, and Schuster, 2000; Lesbian AIDS Project, 1994; Morrow and Allsworth, 2000; Rose, 1993; Stevens, 1994.
65. Lemp, Jones, Kellogg, Nieri, Anderson, Withum, Katz, 1995; Lesbian AIDS Project, 1994; Raiteri et al., 1994; Stevens, 1994.
66. Richardson, 2000.
67. Loue and Mendez, 2006.
68. Ward, 2004; cf. Román, 1995.
69. Richardson, 2000.
70. Loue and Mendez, 2006.

CHAPTER 9

1. Ryan, 1976, p. 10.
2. Ryan, 1976, p. 5.
3. Farmer et al., 2006, p. 449; italics in original.
4. Farmer et al., 2006; Gilligan, 1997.
5. Hudson, 2005; Kelly, 2006.
6. Elliott, 2000.
7. Lillie-Blanton et al., 1993.
8. Williams and Collins, 2001.
9. Latkin and Curry, 2003.
10. Harkness, Newman, and Salkever, 2004.
11. Link and Phelan, 2001.
12. Hogan, 2002.
13. Drake and Wallach, 2000; Drake et al., 2001.
14. Drake et al., 2001.
15. Weisner and Schmidt, 1992.
16. Ramlow et al., 1997.
17. Polak and Warner, 1996.
18. Clark et al., 1998; Dean and Dolan, 1991; Rogers et al., 1995.
19. Hackbarth, Silvestri, and Cosper, 1995; Maxwell and Jacobson, 1989; Moore, Williams, and Qualls, 1996; Rabow and Watt, 1982.
20. Alaniz et al., 1996.
21. Gruenewald, Ponicki, and Holder, 1993; Millar and Gruenewald, 1997.
22. Bernstein et al., 2007.
23. Hill and Angel, 2005.
24. Jacobson, Robinson, and Bluthenthal, 2007.
25. Public and private child welfare institutions in Cleveland have a long history of discrimination against minority children and families. Racial segregation of orphanages and the housing of minority children in dangerous public detention facilities continued into the 1990s (Morton,

2000). Research suggests that the conditions of families receiving welfare in Cuyahoga County, Ohio, have deteriorated since the implementation of welfare reform (Wells et al., 2003).

26. Research findings suggest that only a small proportion of women use substances while they are pregnant. Data derived from the National Household Survey on Drug Abuse (NHSDA) conducted by the Substance Abuse and Mental Health Services Agency (SAMHSA) indicate that, for the years 2002 and 2003, 4.3 percent of pregnant women ages fifteen to forty-four ingested illicit drugs during the month prior to the study interview, compared to 10.4 percent of non-pregnant women in the same age range (Office of Applied Statistics, 2005). A substantially smaller proportion of the pregnant women consumed alcohol (9.8 percent) and engaged in binge drinking (4.1 percent) compared to their non-pregnant counterparts (53.0 percent and 23.2 percent, respectively). The effects of maternal substance use on the fetus during its development and on the child after its birth vary significantly, depending on the substance used and the timing and extent of that use.
27. Brewer, 2004.
28. Hemmens et al., 2002.
29. Ryan, 1976; Wahl, 1995; Wahl, Wood, and Richards, 2002.
30. Herbst et al., 2007; Nyamathi et al., 1994; Villarruel, Jemmott, and Jemmott, 2006.
31. Herbst et al., 2007.
32. Longshore, Stein, and Anglin, 1996.
33. Mishra, Sanudo, and Connor, 2004.
34. Johnson-Massotti et al., 2003.
35. Johnson-Massotti et al., 2003, p. 31.
36. Norton et al., 2009.
37. Carey et al., 2004; Kelly, 1997; Deren et al., 2005.
38. Alegría et al., 2006; Herbst et al., 2007; Holtgrave et al., 1995; Kelly, 1997; Vega and Alegría, 2001; Vega and Lopez, 2001; Weinhardt, Carey, and Carey, 1998.
39. A number of scholars have noted the need for mental health interventions at the level of the community in addition to the usual individual-level approach (Wells et al., 2004) and the transfer of behavioral research technology to community programs (Kalichman et al., 1997). Such efforts, however, do not address the structural elements that are deleterious to individuals' mental well-being and that impede positive behavioral change.
40. McClure, Laibson, Loewenstein, and Cohen, 2004.
41. Kelly (2006) has argued that people with severe mental illness are subject to structural violence and a denial of their rights because of the lack of power among mental health interest groups; the systematic exclusion of mentally ill people from various domains of social, civic, and political life; the difficulties experienced by mentally ill people in identifying and articulating their own needs; and their lack of knowledge with respect to alternative scenarios for their lives.

References

Abad, V., and Suarez, J. (1975). Machismo and alcoholism among Puerto Ricans. In M. E. Chafetz (Ed.). *Proceedings of the Fourth Annual Alcoholism Conference of the National Institute on Alcohol Abuse and Alcoholism* (pp. 282–94). Rockville, MD: National Institute on Alcohol Abuse and Alcoholism.

Adler, P. S. (1975). The transitional experience: An alternative view of culture shock. *Journal of Humanistic Psychology, 15(4)*, 13–23.

Ajzen, I. (1991). The theory of planned behavior. *Organizational Behavior and Human Decision Making Processes, 50*, 179–11.

Akutsu, P. D., Snowden, L. R., and Organista, K. C. (1996). Referral patterns to ethnic specific and mainstream programs for ethnic minorities and whites. *Journal of Counseling Psychology, 43*, 56–64.

Alaniz, M. L., Parker, R. N., Gallegos, A., and Cartmill, R. S. (1996). *Alcohol outlet density and Mexican American youth violence: Final progress report.* Inter-University Program for Latino Research, Ford Foundation.

Aldarondo, E., Kantor, G., and Jasinski, J. L. (2002). A risk marker analysis of wife assault in Latino families. *Violence against Women, 8(4)*, 429–54.

Alegría, M., Canino, G., Ríos, R., Vera, M., Calderón, J., Rusch, D., and Ortega, A. N. (2002). Inequalities in the use of specialty mental health services among Latinos, African Americans, and non-Latino whites. *Psychiatric Services, 53(12)*, 1547–55.

Alegría, M., Chatterji, P., Wells, K., Cao, Z., Chen, C., Takeuchi, D., et al. (2008). Disparity in depression treatment among racial and ethnic minority populations in the United States. *Psychiatric Services, 59(11)*, 1264–72.

Alegría, M., Page, J., Hansen, H., Cauce, A., Robles, R., Blanco, C., et al. (2006). Improving drug treatment services for Hispanics: Research gaps and scientific opportunities. *Drug and Alcohol Dependence, 84*, 76–84.

Allen, J. G., Coyne, L., and Console, P. (1997). Dissociative detachment relates to psychotic symptoms and personality decompensation. *Comprehensive Psychiatry, 38*, 327–34.

Allen, M., Emmers-Sommer, T., and Crowell, T. L. (2002). Couples negotiating safer-sex behaviors: A meta-analysis of the impact of conversation and gender. In M. Allen, R. W. Preiss, B. M. Gayle, and N. A. Burrell (Eds.). *Interpersonal communication research: Advances through meta-analysis* (pp. 263–79). Mahwah, NJ: Erlbaum.

Altman, D. G., Schooler, C., and Basil, M. D. (1991). Alcohol and cigarette advertising on billboards. *Health*

Education Research: Theory and Practice, 6(4), 487–90.

Alvidrez, J. (1999). Ethnic variations in mental health attitudes and service use among low-income African-American, Latina, and European American young women. *Community Mental Health Journal, 35(6)*, 515–30.

Amaro, H. (1988). Considerations of prevention of HIV infection among Hispanic women. *Psychology of Women Quarterly, 12*, 429–43.

American College of Physicians. (2004). Racial and ethnic disparities in health care. *Annals of Internal Medicine, 141(3)*, 226–32.

American Psychiatric Association. (2000). *Diagnostic and statistical manual of mental disorders, fourth edition, text revision (DSM-IV-TR).* Washington, DC: American Psychiatric Association.

Anderson, R. N., and Smith, B. L. (2005). Deaths: Leading causes for 2002. *National Vital Statistics Report, 53(17)*, 51, table 2. Retrieved from *www.cdc.gov/nchs/data/nvsr/nvsr53/nvsr53_17.pdf.*

Angermeyer, M. C., and Matschinger, H. (2003). The stigma of mental illness: Effects of labeling on public attitudes towards people with mental disorder. *Acta Psychiatrica Scandinavica, 108*, 304–9.

Arata, C. M. (1999). Coping with rape: The roles of prior sexual abuse and attributions of blame. *Journal of Interpersonal Violence, 14*, 62–78.

Arredondo, P., Bordes, V., and Paniagua, F. A. (2007). Mexicans, Mexican Americans, Caribbean, and other Latin Americans. In A. J. Marsalla, J. L. Johnson, P. Watson, and J. Gryczynski (Eds.). *Ethnocultural perspectives on disaster and trauma* (pp. 299–320). New York: Springer.

Arriola, K. R. J., Louden, T., Doldren, M. A., and Fortenberry, R. M. (2005). A meta-analysis of the relationship of child sexual abuse to HIV risk behavior among women. *Child Abuse and Neglect, 29*, 725–46.

Aruffo, J., Cloverdale, J. H., Chacko, R. C., and Dworkin, R. J. (1990). Knowledge about AIDS among women psychiatric outpatients. *Hospital and Community Psychiatry, 41*, 326–28.

Atdjian, S., and Vega, W. (2005). Disparities in mental health treatment in U.S. racial and ethnic minority groups: Implications for psychiatrists. *Psychiatric Services, 56(12)*, 1600–1602.

Baca Zinn, M. (1982). Chicano men and masculinity. *Journal of Ethnic Studies, 10*, 20–44.

Baker, S. S. (2002). *Understanding mainland Puerto Rican poverty*. Philadelphia: Temple University Press.

Barrera, V., and Bielby, D. D. (2004). Places, faces, and other familiar things: The cultural experience of telenovela viewing among Latinos in the United States. *Journal of Popular Culture, 34(4)*, 1–18.

Barrio, C., Yamada, A. M., Hough, R. L., Hawthorne, W., Garcia, R., and Jeste, D. (2003). Ethnic disparities in use of public mental health case management services among patients with schizophrenia. *Psychiatric Services, 54(9)*, 1264–70.

Bartels, S. J. (2003). Improving the system of care for older adults with mental illness in the United States: Findings and recommendations for the President's New Freedom Commission on Mental Health. *American Journal of Geriatric Psychiatry, 11*, 486–97.

Bauer, M. S., and McBride, L. (2003). *Structured group psychotherapy for bipolar disorder: The Life Goals Program*, 2nd ed. New York: Springer.

Bean, F., and Tienda, M. (1988). *Hispanic population in the U.S.* New York: Russell Sage Foundation.

Bechara, A., and Damasio, H. (2002). Decision-making and addiction (part I): Impaired activation of somatic states in substance dependent individuals when pondering decisions with negative future consequences. *Neuropsychologia, 39*, 376–89.

Becker, D. R., Drake, R. E., Bond, G. R.,

Xie, H., Dain, B. J., and Harrison, K. (1998). Job terminations among patients with severe mental illness participating in supported employment. *Community Mental Health Journal, 34*, 71–82.

Becker, H. (1963). *The outsiders*. Glencoe, IL: Free Press.

Bellack, A. S., Mueser, K. T., Gingerich, S., and Agresta, J. (1997). *Social skills training for schizophrenia: A step-by-step guide*. New York: Guilford Press.

Belle, D. (Ed.). (1982). *Lives in stress: Women and depression*. Beverly Hills, CA: Sage.

Benavides, J. (1992). Mujeres rule the roosters. *Santa Barbara News Press*, Oct. 17, B1.

Bender, E. (2006). Data confirm MH crisis growing in U.S. prisons. *Psychiatric News, 41(20)*, 6–26.

Bernal, G., and Alvarez, A. (1983). Culture and class in the study of families. In C. Falicov (Ed.). *Cultural perspectives in family therapy* (pp. 33–50). Rockville, MD: Aspen.

Bernstein, K. T., Galea, S., Ahern, J., Tracy, M., and Vlahov, D. (2007). The built environment and alcohol consumption in urban neighborhoods. *Drug and Alcohol Dependence, 91*, 244–52.

Bifulco, A., and Moran, P. (1998). *Wednesday's child: Research into women's experience of neglect and abuse in childhood and adult depression*. London: Routledge.

Biglan, A., Metzler, C. W., Wirt, R., Ary, D. V., Noell, J., Ochs, L., et al. (1990). Social and behavioral factors associated with high-risk sexual behavior among adolescents. *Journal of Behavioral Medicine, 13*, 245–61.

Blank, M. B., Mandell, D. S., Aiken, L., and Hadley, T. R. (2002). Co-occurrence of HIV and serious mental illness among Medicaid recipients. *Psychiatric Services, 53(7)*, 868–73.

Bond, G. R., Resnick, S. G., Drake, R. E., Xie, H., McHugo, G. J., and Bebout, R. R. (2001). Does competitive employment improve motivational outcomes for people with severe mental illness? *Journal of Clinical and Consulting Psychology, 69(3)*, 489–501.

Borjas, G. (1985). Jobs and employment for Hispanics. In P. San Juan Cafferty and W. C. McCready (Eds.). *Hispanics in the United States*. New Brunswick, NJ: Transaction.

Borowsky, S. J., Robernstein, L. V., Meredith, L. S., Camp, P., Jackson-Triche, M., and Wells, K. B. (2000). Who is at risk of nondetection of mental health problems in primary care? *Journal of General Internal Medicine, 15*, 381–88.

Bourgois, P. (1995). *In search of respect: Selling crack in El Barrio*. New York: Cambridge University Press.

Bowers, B., Joyce, M., and Esmond, S. (1996). *Quality care: The perspectives of individuals with physical disabilities and their caregivers*. Madison: University of Wisconsin–Madison.

Brabin, L. (2001). Hormonal markers of susceptibility to sexually transmitted infections: Are we taking them seriously? *British Medical Journal, 323*, 394–95.

Bravo, M. (1989). *Las redes de apoyo social y las situaciones de desastre: Estudio de la población adulto en P.R.* Rio Piedras: University of Puerto Rico.

Brewer, R. M. (2004). Family structure. In G. Mink and A. O'Connor (Eds.). *Poverty in the United States: An encyclopedia of history, politics, and policy* (pp. 306–8). Santa Barbara, CA: ABL-CLIO.

Briere, J. (2002). Treating adult survivors of severe childhood abuse and neglect: Further development of an integrative model. In L. Berliner, J. E. B. Myers, J. Briere, C. T. Hendrix, C. Jenny, and T. Reid (Eds.). *The APSAC handbook on child maltreatment*, 2nd ed. (pp. 175–204). Newbury Park, CA: Sage.

Briere, J., and Elliott, D. M. (2003). Prevalence and psychological sequelae of self-reported childhood physical and sexual abuse in a general population sample of men and women. *Child Abuse and Neglect, 27*, 1205–22.

Briggs, L. (1998). Discourses of "forced sterilization" in Puerto Rico: The problem with the speaking subaltern. *Differences: A Journal of Feminist Cultural Studies, 10(2)*, 30–66.

Brockington, I. F., Hall, P., Levings, J., and Murphy, C. (1993). The community's tolerance of the mentally ill. *British Journal of Psychiatry, 162*, 93–99.

Brookings Institution. (2003). *Cleveland in focus: A profile from census 2000.* Washington, DC: Brookings Institution. Retrieved May 22, 2009, from *www.brookings.edu/reports/2003/11_livingcities_cleveland.aspx.*

Brown, L. K., Danovsky, M. B., Lourie, K. J., DiClemente, R. J., and Ponton, L. E. (1997). Adolescents with psychiatric disorders and the risk of HIV. *Journal of the American Academy of Child and Adolescent Psychiatry, 36*, 1609–17.

Brown, L. K., Houck, C. D., Hadley, W. S., and Lescano, C. M. (2005). Self-cutting and sexual risk among adolescents in intensive psychiatric treatment. *Psychiatric Services, 56(2)*, 216–18.

Bruce, M. L., Wells, K. B., Miranda, J., Lewis, L., and Gonzalez, J. J. (2002). Barriers to reducing burden of affective disorders. *Mental Health Services Research, 4(4)*, 187–97.

Bruinius, H. (2006). *Better for all the world: The secret history of forced sterilization and America's quest for racial purity*. New York: Alfred A. Knopf.

Buckley, P., Thompson, P., Way, L., and Meltzer, H. (1994). Substance abuse among patients with treatment-resistant schizophrenia: Characteristics and implications for clozapine therapy. *American Journal of Psychiatry, 151*, 385–89.

Buell, G. J., and Anthony, W. A. (1973). Demographic characteristics as predictors of recidivism and post-hospital employment. *Journal of Counseling Psychiatry, 20*, 361–65.

Bunt, L. (1988). Music therapy: An introduction. *Psychology of Music, 16*, 3–9.

Burgess, E. W., Locke, H. J., and Thomes, M. M. (1963). *The family: From institution to companionship*, 3rd ed. New York: American Book Company.

Burns, T., Creed, F., Fahy, T., Thompson, S., Tyrer, P., and White, I. (1999). Intensive versus standard case management for severe psychotic illness: A randomized trial. *Lancet, 353*, 2185–89.

Bushman, B., and Cooper, H. (1990). Effects of alcohol on human aggression: An integrative research review. *Psychological Bulletin, 107(3)*, 341–54.

Campbell, J. (1989). Women's response to sexual abuse in intimate relationships. *Health Care for Women International, 10*, 335–46.

Campos, R., and Bonilla, F. (1976). Industrialization and migration: Some effects on the Puerto Rican working class. *Latin American Perspectives, 3*, 79.

Capitanio, J. P., and Herek, G. M. (1999). AIDS-related stigma and attitudes toward injecting drug users among black and white Americans. *American Behavioral Scientist, 42(7)*, 1148–61.

Carey, M. P., Carey, K. B., and Kalichman, S. C. (1997). Risk for human immunodeficiency virus (HIV) infection among persons with severe mental illnesses. *Clinical Psychology Review, 17*, 271–91.

Carey, M. P., Carey, K. B., Maisto, S. A., Gordon, C. M., Schroder, K. E. E., and Vanable, P. A. (2004). Reducing HIV-risk behavior among adults receiving outpatient psychiatric treatment: Results from a randomized controlled trial. *Journal of Consulting and Clinical Psychology, 72(2)*, 252–68.

Carey, M. P., Carey, K. B., Weinhardt, L. S., and Gordon, C. M. (1997a). Behavioral risk for HIV infection among adults with a severe and persistent mental illness: Patterns and psychological antecedents. *Community Mental Health Journal, 33*, 133–42.

Carey, M. P., Carey, K. B., Weinhardt, L. S., and Gordon, C. M. (1997b). Documented behavioral risk for human immunodeficiency virus (HIV) infection among seriously mentally ill outpatients. *Community Mental Health Journal, 33,* 133–42.

Carling, P. (1995). *Return to community: Building support systems for people with psychiatric disabilities.* New York: Guilford.

Caron, J., Tempier, R., Mercier, C., and Leouffre, P. (1998). Components of social support and quality of life in severely mentally ill, low income individuals and a general population Group. *Community Mental Health Journal, 34(5),* 459–75.

Casas, J. M., Wagenheim, B. R., Banchero, R., and Mendoza-Romero, J. (1994). Hispanic masculinity: Myth or psychological schema meriting clinical consideration. *Hispanic Journal of Behavioral Sciences, 16(3),* 315–31.

Castle, D. J., and Morgan, V. (2008) Epidemiology. In K. T. Mueser and D. V. Jeste (Eds.). *Clinical handbook of schizophrenia* (pp. 14–24). New York: Guilford Press.

Caton, C. L. M., Shrout, P. E., Eagle, P. F., Opler, L. A., Felix, A., and Dominguez, B. (1994). Risk factors for homelessness among schizophrenic men: A case-control study. *American Journal of Public Health, 84,* 265–70.

Celentano, D. D., Latimore, A. D., and Mehta, S. H. (2008). Variations in sexual risks in drug users: Emerging themes in a behavioral context. *Current HIV/AIDS Reports, 5,* 212–18.

Center on Budget and Policy Priorities. (1988). *Shortchanged: Recent developments in Hispanic poverty, income and employment.* Washington, DC: Center on Budget and Policy Priorities.

Centers for Disease Control and Prevention. (2009). HIV prevalence estimates—United States, 2006. *Journal of the American Medical Association, 301(1),* 27–29.

Centers for Disease Control and Prevention. (2008). *HIV/AIDS among Hispanics,* April. Retrieved August 13, 2008, from *www.cdc.gov/hiv/hispanics/resources/factsheets/hispanic.htm.*

Centers for Disease Control and Prevention. (2006). *HIV/AIDS among Hispanics,* June.

Centers for Disease Control and Prevention. (2003a). Advancing HIV prevention: New strategies for a changing epidemic—United States, 2003. *Morbidity and Mortality Weekly Report, 52(15),* 329–32.

Centers for Disease Control and Prevention. (2003b). HIV testing—United States, 2001. *Morbidity and Mortality Weekly Report, 52(23),* 540–45.

Chartier, M. J., Walker, J. R., and Naimark, B. (2007). Childhood abuse, adult health, and health care utilization: Results from a representative community sample. *American Journal of Epidemiology, 165,* 1031–38.

Chenault, L. R. (1970). *The Puerto Rican migrant in New York City.* New York: Russell and Russell.

Chow, J. C.-C., Jaffee, K., and Snowden, L. (2003). Racial/ethnic disparities in the use of mental health services in poverty areas. *American Journal of Public Health, 93(5),* 792–97.

Clark, R. E., Dain, B. J., Xie, H., Becker, D. R., and Drake, R. E. (1998). The economic benefits of supported employment for persons with mental illness. *Journal of Mental Health Policy and Economics, 1,* 63–71.

Clark, R. E., and Drake, R. E. (1994). Expenditures of time and money by families of people with severe mental illness and substance use disorders. *Community Mental Health Journal, 30(2),* 145–63.

Cleveland Department of Public Health. (2009). The number of persons living with HIV/AIDS (i.e. prevalence) in Cleveland neighborhoods (statistical planning areas) as of December 31, 2008. Retrieved April 20, 2009 from *clevelandhealth.info/Members/db/export09/hivprevspa2008.*

Cleveland Department of Public Health. (2008). *Cleveland only HIV/AIDS prevalence report: Reported persons living with HIV/AIDS as of December 31, 2007, final report.*

Cleveland Department of Public Health. (2007). *STD report for Cuyahoga County, 2004–2005.*

Cleveland Department of Public Health. (2006). *HIV/AIDS report for Cleveland.* May 24.

Cloitre, M., Tardiff, K., Marzuk, P., Leon, A. C., and Potera, L. (1996). Childhood abuse and subsequent sexual assault among female inpatients. *Journal of Traumatic Stress, 9*, 473–82.

Collins, P. Y. (2001). Dual taboos: Sexuality and women with severe mental illness in South Africa; Perceptions of mental health care providers. *AIDS and Behavior, 5(2)*, 151–61.

Connell, R. W. (1987). *Gender and power: Society, the person, and sexual politics.* Palo Alto, CA: Stanford University Press.

Coohey, C. (2001). The relationship between familism and child maltreatment in Latino and Anglo families. *Child Maltreatment, 6(2)*, 130–42.

Cook, J. (2005). *Executive summary of findings from the employment intervention demonstration program.* Retrieved from *www.psych.uic.edu/eidp/eidpubs.htm.*

Cooley, C. (1902). *Human nature and the social order.* New York: Scribner.

Cournos, F., Empfield, M., Horwath, E., McKinnon, K., Meyer, I., Schrage, H., Currie, C., and Agosin, B. (1991). HIV seroprevalence among patients admitted to two psychiatric hospitals. *American Journal of Psychiatry, 148*, 1225–30.

Cournos, F., Horwath, E., Guido, J. R., McKinnon, K., and Hopkins, N. (1994). HIV-1 infection at two public psychiatric hospitals in New York City. *AIDS Care, 6*, 443–52.

Cournos, F., and McKinnon, K. (1997). HIV seroprevalence among people with severe mental illness in the United States: A critical review. *Clinical Psychology Review, 17*, 259–69.

Craine, L. S., Henson, C. E., Colliver, J. A., and MacLean, D. G. (1988). Prevalence of a history of sexual abuse among female psychiatric patients in a state hospital system. *Hospital and Community Psychiatry, 39*, 300–304.

Cramer, J. A., and Rosenheck, P. (1998). Compliance with medication regimens for mental and physical disorders. *Psychiatric Services, 49*, 196–201.

Cromwell, R. E., and Ruiz, R. A. (1979). The myth of macho dominance in decision making within Mexican and Chicano families. *Hispanic Journal of Behavioral Sciences, 1*, 355–73.

Cruz, D., and Serrano-García, I. (1997). La relación entre la percepción de moralidad y las prácticas sexuales de alto riesgo en mujeres puertorriqueñas [The relationship between perceptions of morality and high-risk sexual practices in Puerto Rican women]. Paper presented at the Interamerican Congress of Psychology, Sao Paolo, Brazil. Cited in Ortiz-Torres, B., Serrano-García, I., and Torres-Burgos, N. (2000). Subverting culture: Promoting HIV/AIDS prevention among Puerto Rican and Dominican women. *American Journal of Community Psychology, 28(6)*, 859–81.

Cruz, J. E. (1998). *Identity and power: Puerto Rican politics and the challenge of ethnicity.* Philadelphia: Temple University Press.

Cuffel, B. J. (1996). Comorbid substance use disorder: Prevalence, patterns of use, and course. *New Directions for Mental Health Services, 70*, 93–106.

Cunningham, I. (1998). An innovative HIV/AIDS research and education program in Puerto Rico. *SIECUS Report, 26*, 18–20.

Cunningham, K., Wolbert, R., and Brockmeier, M. B. (2000). Moving beyond the illness: Factors contributing to gaining and maintaining employment. *American Journal of Community Psychology, 28*, 481–94.

Cunningham, R. M., Stiffman, A. R., Dore,

P., and Earls, F. (1994). The association of physical and sexual abuse with HIV risk behaviors in adolescence and young adulthood: Implications for public health. *Child Abuse and Neglect, 18*, 233–45.

Cunradi, C. B., Cateano, R., and Schafer, J. (2002). Socioeconomic predictors of intimate partner violence among white, black, and Hispanic couples in the United States. *Journal of Family Violence, 17(4)*, 377–88.

Daly, R. (2006). Prison mental health crisis continues to grow. *Psychiatric News, 41(20)*, 1–5.

Daumit, G. L., Crum, R. M., Guallar, E., Powe, N. R., Primm, A. B., Steinwachs, D. M., et al. (2003). Outpatient prescriptions for atypical antipsychotics for African Americans, Hispanics, and Whites in the United States. *Archives of General Psychiatry, 60*, 121–28.

Davenport, Y., Zahn-Waxler, C., Adland, M., and Mayfield, A. (1984). Early child-rearing practices in families with a manic-depressive parent. *American Journal of Psychiatry, 141*, 230–35.

De La Cancela, V. (1986). A critical analysis of Puerto Rican machismo: Implications for clinical practice. *Psychotherapy, 23(2)*, 291–96.

Dean, D. H., and Dolan, R. C. (1991). Assessing the role of vocational rehabilitation in disability policy. *Journal of Policy Analysis and Management, 10*, 568–87.

Delgado, M. (1977). Puerto Rican spiritualism and the social work profession. *Social Casework, Oct.*, 451–58.

Demo, D. H., Small, S. A., and Savin-Williams, R. C. (1987). Family relations and the self-esteem of adolescents and their parents. *Journal of Marriage and the Family, 49*, 705–15.

Deren, S., Shedlin, M., Decena, C. U., and Mino, M. (2005). Research challenges to the study of HIV/AIDS among migrant and immigrant Hispanic populations in the United States. *Journal of Urban Health, 82(2: Supp. 3)*, iii13–iii25.

Des Jarlais, D. C., and Semaan, S. (2009). HIV prevention and psychoactive drug use: A research agenda. *Journal of Epidemiology and Community Health, 63*, 191–96.

Devereux, G. (1958). Cultural thought models in primitive and modern psychological theories. *Psychiatry, 21*, 359–74.

Dévieux, J. G., Malow, R., Lerner, B. G., Dyer, J. G., Baptista, L., Lucenko, B., et al. (2007). Triple jeopardy for HIV: Substance using severely mentally ill adults. *Journal of Prevention and Intervention in the Community, 33(1–2)*, 5–18.

Diamant, A. L., Lever, J., and Schuster, M. A. (2000). Lesbians' sexual activities and efforts to reduce risks for sexually transmitted diseases. *Journal of the Gay and Lesbian Medical Association, 4(2)*, 41–48.

Diaz-Guerrero, R. (1955). Neurosis and the Mexican family structure. *American Journal of Psychiatry, 112*, 411–17.

Díaz-Olavarrieta, C., Ellertson, C., Paz, F., Ponce de Leon, S., and Alarcon-Segovia, D. (2002). Prevalence of battery among 1780 outpatients at an internal medical institution in Mexico. *Social Science and Medicine, 55*, 1589–1602.

Dixon, D., Peters, M., and Saul, J. (2003). HIV sexual risk among Puerto Rican women. *Health Care for Women International, 24*, 529–43.

Dixon, D. A., Antoni, M., Peters, M., and Saul, J. (2001). Employment, social support, and HIV sexual-risk behavior in Puerto Rican women. *AIDS and Behavior, 5(4)*, 331–42.

Dixon, L., Haas, G., Weiden, P. J., Sweeney, J., and Frances, A. J. (1991). Drug abuse in schizophrenic patients: Clinical correlates and reasons for use. *American Journal of Psychiatry, 148(2)*, 224–30.

Downar, J., and Kapur, S. (2008). Biological theories. In K. T. Mueser and D. V. Jeste (Eds.). *Clinical handbook of schizophrenia* (pp. 25–34). New York: Guilford Press.

Drake, R. E., Essock, S. M., Shaner, A.,

Carey, K. B., Minkoff, K., Kola, L., et al. (2001). Implementing dual diagnosis services for clients with severe mental illness. *Psychiatric Services, 52(4)*, 469–76.

Drake, R. E., and Wallach, M. A. (2000). Dual diagnosis: 15 years of progress. *Psychiatric Services, 51*, 1126–29.

Driscoll, A. K., Briggs, M. A., Brindis, C. D., and Yankah, E. (2001). Adolescent Latino reproductive health: A review of the literature. *Hispanic Journal of Behavioral Sciences, 23*, 255–326.

Dutton, D. G., and Painter, S. L. (1993). Emotional attachments in abusive relationships: A test of traumatic bonding theory. *Violence and Victims, 8*, 105–20.

Dutton, D. G., and Painter, S. L. (1981). Traumatic bonding: The development of emotional attachments in battered women and other relationships of intermittent abuse. *Victimology: An International Journal, 1*, 139–55.

Edwards, V. J., Holden, G. W., Felitti, V. J., and Anda, R. F. (2003). Relationship between multiple forms of childhood maltreatment and adult mental health in community respondents: Results from the Adverse Childhood Experiences Study. *American Journal of Psychiatry, 160(8)*, 1453–60.

El-Bassel, N., Witte, S. S., Wada, T., Gilbert, L., and Wallace, J. (2001). Correlates of partner violence among female street-based sex workers: Substance abuse, history of childhood abuse, and HIV risks. *AIDS Patient Care and STDs, 15*, 41–51.

Elliott, M. (2000). The stress process in neighborhood context. *Health Place, 6*, 287–99.

Ellman, L. M., and Cannon, T. D. (2008). Environmental pre- and perinatal influences in etiology. In K. T. Mueser and D. V. Jeste (Eds.). *Clinical handbook of schizophrenia* (pp. 65–73). New York: Guilford Press.

Empfield, M., Cournos, F., Meyer, I., McKinnon, K., Horwath, E., Silver, M., Schrage, H., and Herman, R. (1993). HIV seroprevalence among homeless patients admitted to a psychiatric inpatient unit. *American Journal of Psychiatry, 150*, 47–52.

Erikson, E. (1968). *Identity, youth, and crisis.* New York: Norton.

Farmer, P. E. (2004). An anthropology of structural violence. *Current Anthropology, 45(3)*, 305–25.

Farmer, P. E., Nizeye, B., Stulac, S., and Keshvajee, S. (2006). Structural violence and clinical medicine. *PLoS Medicine, 3(10)*, e449. doi:10.1371/journal.pmed.0030449.

Faulkner, I. (2003). Good girl or flirt girl: Latinas' definition of sex and sexual relationships. *Hispanic Journal of Behavioral Sciences, 25(2)*, 174–200.

Favazza, A. R., and Conterio, K. (1988). The plight of chronic self-mutilators. *Community Mental Health, 24*, 22–30.

Fellitti, V. (1991). Long-term medical consequences of incest, rape, and molestation. *Southern Medical Journal, 84*, 328–31.

Fernández-Marina, R. (1961). The Puerto Rican syndrome. *Psychiatry, 24*, 79–82.

Finkelhor, D., and Browne, A. (1985). The traumatic impact of child sexual abuse: A conceptualization. *American Journal of Orthopsychiatry, 55(4)*, 530–41.

Finkelhor, D., Hotaling, G., Lewis, I. A., and Smith, C. (1990). Sexual abuse in a national survey of adult men and women: Prevalence, characteristics, and risk factors. *Child Abuse and Neglect, 14*, 19–28.

Finn, P. R., Justus, A., Mazas, C., and Steinmetz, J. E. (1999). Working memory, executive processes, and the effects of alcohol on go/no-go learning: Testing a model of behavioral regulation in impulsivity. *Psychopharmacology, 146*, 465–72.

Fiscella, K., Franks, P., Doecher, M. P., and Saver, B. G. (2002). Disparities in health care by race, ethnicity, and language among the insured: Findings from a national sample. *Medical Care, 40(1)*, 52–59.

Fisher, J. D., Fisher, W. A., Williams, S. S.,

and Malloy, T. E. (1994). Empirical tests of an information-motivation-behavioral skills model of AIDS preventive behavior. *Health Psychologist, 13*, 228–50.

Fitchett, G., Burton, L. A., and Sivan, A. B. (1997). The religious needs and resources of psychiatric patients. *Journal of Nervous and Mental Disease, 185*, 320–26.

Fitzpatrick, J. P. (1987). *Puerto Rican Americans: The meaning of migration to the mainland.* Englewood Cliffs, NJ: Prentice-Hall.

Fleuridas, C., Crevy, K., and Vela, E. (1997). Sexual risk-taking in college students and functional families of origin. *Family Systems and Health, 15*, 185–202.

Folsom, D. P., Hawthorne, W., Lindamer, L., Gilmer, T., Bailey, A., Golshan, S., et al. (2005). Prevalence and risk factors for homelessness and utilization of mental health services among 10,340 patients with serious mental illness in a large public mental health system. *American Journal of Psychiatry, 162(2)*, 370–76.

Foster, R. H., and Goa, K. L. (1999). Olanzapine: A pharmacoeconomic review of its use in schizophrenia. *Pharmacoeconomics, 15*, 611–40.

Francell, C., Conn, V., and Gray, D. (1988). Families' perceptions of burden of care for chronic mentally ill relatives. *Hospital and Community Psychiatry, 39*, 1296–300.

Frankel, K. A., and Harmon, R. J. (1996). Depressed mothers: They don't always look as bad as they feel. *Journal of the American Academy of Child and Adolescent Psychiatry, 35*, 289–98.

Fraser, R. T., and Shrey, D. E. (1986). Perceived barriers to job placement revisited: Toward practical solutions. *Journal of Rehabilitation*, Autumn, 26–29.

Fromme, K., D'Amico, E. J., and Katz, E. C. (1999). Intoxicated sexual risk taking: An expectancy or cognitive impairment explanation? *Journal of Studies on Alcohol, 24*, 313–19.

Gagnon, J. H., and Simon, W. (1973). *Sexual conduct: The social sources of human sexuality*. Piscataway, NJ: Aldine.

Galanti, G. A. (2003). The Hispanic family and male-female relationships: An overview. *Journal of Transcultural Nursing, 14*, 180–85.

Galtung, J. (1969). Violence, peace, and peace research. *Journal of Peace Research, 6*, 167–91.

Gandhi, D. H., Bogrov, M. U., Osher, F. C., and Myers, C. P. (2003). A comparison of the patterns of drug use among patients with and without severe mental illness. *American Journal of Addictions, 12*, 424–31.

Geanellos, R. (2003). Understanding the need for personal space boundary restoration in women-client survivors of intrafamilial childhood sexual abuse. *International Journal of Mental Health Nursing, 12*, 186–93.

Gearon, J. S., and Bellack, A. S. (1999). Women with schizophrenia and co-occurring substance use disorders: An increased risk for violent victimization and HIV. *Community Mental Health, 35*, 401–19.

Geddes, J., Freemantle, N., Harrison, P., and Bebbington, P. (2000). Atypical antipsychotics in the treatment of schizophrenia: Systematic overview and meta-regression analysis. *British Medical Journal, 321*, 1371–76.

George, W. G. H., Davis, K. C., Norris, J., Herman, J. R., Stoner, S. I., Schacht, R. L., et al. (2007). Indirect effects of acute alcohol intoxication in sexual risk-taking: The roles of subjective and physiological sexual arousal. *Archives of Sexual Behavior* (e-pub ahead of print).

Gherovici, P. (2003). *The Puerto Rican syndrome*. New York: Other Press.

Gilligan, C. (1982). *In a different voice*. Cambridge, MA: Harvard University Press.

Gilligan, J. (1997). *Violence: Reflections on a national epidemic*. New York: Vintage Books.

Ginsburg, G. P. (1988). Rules, scripts, and prototypes in personal relationships. In S. W. Duck (Ed.). *Handbook of personal relationships* (pp. 23–39). London: Wiley.

Giraldo, O. (1972). El machismo como

fenómeno psicocultural [Machismo as a psychocultural phenomenon]. *Revista Mexicana de Psicología, 4*, 295–309.

Gladstone, G. L., Parker, G. B., Mitchell, P. B., Malhi, G. S., Wilhelm, K., and Austin, M.-P. (2004). Implications of childhood trauma for depressed women: An analysis of pathways from childhood sexual abuse to deliberate self-harm and revictimization. *American Journal of Psychiatry, 161(8)*, 1417–25.

Glatt, S. J. (2008). Genetics. In K. T. Mueser and D. V. Jeste (Eds.). *Clinical handbook of schizophrenia* (pp. 55–64). New York: Guilford Press.

Glazer, N., and Moynihan, D. P. (1963). *Beyond the melting pot*. Cambridge, MA: Harvard-MIT Press.

Glenn, S. W., and Parsons, O. A. (1992). Neuropsychological efficiency measures in male and female alcoholics. *Journal of Studies on Alcohol, 53*, 546–52.

Goffman, E. (1963). *Stigma: Notes on the management of spoiled identity*. New York: Touchstone.

Gold, C., Heldal, T. O., Dahle, T., and Wigram, T. (2005). Music therapy for schizophrenia or schizophrenia-like illnesses. *Cochrane Database Systems Review, 2*, CD004025.

Gonzalez, A. (1982). Sex roles of the traditional Mexican American family: A comparison of Chicano and Anglo students' attitudes. *Journal of Cross-Cultural Psychology, 13*, 330–39.

Good, B. J. (1977). The heart of what's the matter: The semantics of illness in Iran. *Culture, Medicine, and Psychiatry, 1*, 25–58.

Goodman, L. A., Dutton, M. A., and Harris, M. (1995). Episodically homeless women with serious mental illness: Prevalence of physical and sexual assault. *American Journal of Orthopsychiatry, 65*, 468–78.

Goodman, L. A., and Fallot, R. D. (1998). HIV risk-behavior in poor urban women with serious mental illness: Association with childhood physical and sexual abuse. *American Journal of Orthopsychiatry, 68*, 73–83.

Goodman, L. A., Rosenberg, S. D., Mueser, K. T., and Drake, R. E. (1997). Physical and sexual assault history in women with severe mental illness: Prevalence, correlates, treatment, and future research directions. *Schizophrenia Bulletin, 23*, 685–96.

Goodman, L. A., Salyers, M. P., Mueser, K. T., Rosenberg, S. D., Swartz, M., Essock, S. M., et al. (2001). Recent victimization in men and women with severe mental illness: Prevalence and correlates. *Journal of Traumatic Stress, 14*, 615–32.

Goodman, S., Adamson, L., Riniti, J., and Cole, S. (1994). Mothers' expressed attitudes: Associations with maternal depression and children's self-esteem and psychopathology. *Journal of the American Academy of Child and Adolescent Psychiatry, 33*, 1265–74.

Goodwin, F. K., and Jamison, K. R. (1990). *Manic-depressive illness*. New York: Oxford University Press.

Grant, I. (1987). Alcohol and the brain: Neuropsychological correlates. *Journal of Consulting and Clinical Psychology, 55*, 310–24.

Grant, I., and Judd, L. L. (1976). Neuropsychological and EEG disturbances in polydrug-users. *American Journal of Psychiatry, 133*, 1039–42.

Gruenewald, P. J., Ponicki, W. R., and Holder, H. D. (1993). The relationship of outlet densities to alcohol consumption: A time-series cross-sectional analysis. *Alcoholism: Clinical and Experimental Research, 17(1)*, 38–47.

Guarnaccia, P. J. (1993). Ataques de nervios in Puerto Rico: Culture-bound syndrome or popular illness? *Medical Anthropology, 15*, 157–70.

Guarnaccia, P. J., Canino, G., Rubio-Stipec, M., and Bravo, M. (1993). The prevalence of ataques de nervios in the Puerto Rico Disaster Study: The role of culture in psychiatric epidemiology. *Journal of Nervous and Mental Disease, 181*, 157–65.

Guarnaccia, P. J., Lewis-Fernández, R., and

Rivera Marano, M. (2003). Toward a Puerto Rican popular nosology: *Nervios* and *ataque de nervios*. *Culture, Medicine, and Psychiatry, 27*, 339–66.

Guarnaccia, P. J., Parra, P., Deschamps, A., Milstein, G., and Argiles, N. (1992). So Dios quiere: Hispanic families' experiences of caring for a seriously mentally ill family member. *Culture, Medicine, and Psychiatry, 16*, 187–215.

Guarnaccia, P. J., and Rogler, L. (1999). Research on culture bound syndromes: New directions. *American Journal of Psychiatry, 156(9)*, 1322–27.

Guarnaccia, P. J., Rubio-Stipec, M., and Canino, G. (1989). Ataques de nervios in the Puerto Rican Diagnostic Interview Schedule: The impact of cultural categories on psychiatric epidemiology. *Culture, Medicine, and Psychiatry, 13*, 275–95.

Haaken, J. (1993). From Al-Anon to ACOA: Codependence and the reconstruction of caregiving. *Signs, 18(2)*, 321–45.

Hackbarth, D. P., Silvestri, B., and Cosper, W. (1995). Tobacco and alcohol billboards in 50 Chicago neighborhoods: Market segmentation to sell dangerous products to the poor. *Journal of Public Health Policy, 16(2)*, 213–30.

Hall, J. C., Smith, K., and Shimkunas, A. (1966). Employment problems of schizophrenic patients. *American Journal of Psychiatry, 123*, 536–40.

Hamilton, E. B., Jones, M., and Hammen, C. (1993). Maternal interaction style in affective disordered, physically ill, and normal women. *Family Process, 32(3)*, 329–40.

Hammer, J. C., Fisher, J. D., Fitzgerald, P., and Fisher, W. A. (1996). When two heads aren't better than one: AIDS risk behavior in college-age couples. *Journal of Applied Social Psychology, 26*, 375–97.

Handlin, O. (1959). *The newcomers: Negroes and Puerto Ricans in a changing metropolis*. Cambridge, MA: Harvard University Press.

Hansen, H. (2004a). Faith-based treatment for addiction in Puerto Rico. *Journal of the American Medical Association, 291(23)*, 2882.

Hansen, H. (2004b). Faith-based treatments for addiction dominate in Puerto Rico. *Brown University Digest of Addiction Theory and Application, 23(10)*, 4.

Hanson, M., Kramer, T. H., Gross, W., Quintana, J., Li, P., and Asher, R. (1992). AIDS awareness and risk behaviors among dually disordered adults. *AIDS Education and Prevention, 4*, 41–51.

Harkness, J., Newman, S. J., and Salkever, D. (2004). The cost-effectiveness of independent housing for the chronically mentally ill: Do housing and neighborhood features matter? *Health Services Research, 39(5)*, 1341–60.

Harman, J. J., O'Grady, M. A., and Wilson, K. (2009). What you think you know can hurt you: Perceptual biases about HIV risk in intimate relationships. *AIDS Behavior, 13*, 246–47.

Harman, J. S., Edlund, M. J., and Fortney, J. C. (2004). Disparities in the adequacy of depression treatment in the United States. *Psychiatric Services, 55*, 1379–85.

Harper, F. D., and Bruce-Sanford, G. C. (1989). *Counseling techniques: An outline and overview.* Alexandria, VA: Douglass.

Hatters-Friedman, S., and Loue, S. (2007). Incidence and prevalence of intimate partner violence by and against women with severe mental illness. *Journal of Women's Health, 16(4)*, 471–80.

Hayashi, N., Tanabe, Y., Nakagawa, S., Noguchi, M., Iwata, C., Koubuchi, Y., et al. (2002). Effects of group musical therapy on inpatients with chronic psychoses: A controlled study. *Psychiatry and Clinical Neuroscience, 56*, 187–93.

Haywood, T. W., Kravitz, H. M., Grossman, L. S., Cavanaugh, J. L., Jr., Davis, J. M., and Lewis, D. A. (1995). Predicting the "revolving door" phenomenon among patients with schizophrenic, schizoaffective, and affective disorders. *American Journal of Psychiatry, 152*, 856–61.

Hemmens, C., Miller, M., Burton, V. S., and Milner, S. (2002). The consequences of official labels: An examination of the rights lost by the mentally ill and mentally incompetent ten years later. *Community Mental Health Journal, 38*, 129–40.

Herbst, J. H., Kay, L. S., Passin, W. F., Lyles, C. M., Crepaz, N., and Marín, B. V. (2007). HIV/AIDS Prevention Research Synthesis team. A systematic review and meta-analysis of behavioral interventions to reduce HIV risk behaviors of Hispanics in the United States and Puerto Rico. *AIDS Behavior, 11*, 25–47.

Herek, G. M. (1999). AIDS and stigma. *American Behavioral Scientist, 42(7)*, 1106–16.

Herek, G. M., and Capitanio, J. P. (1999). AIDS stigma and sexual prejudice. *American Behavioral Scientist, 42(7)*, 1130–47.

Higgins, E. T., King, G. A., and Mavin, G. H. (1982). Individual construct accessibility and subjective impression and recall. *Journal of Personality and Social Psychology, 73*, 35–47.

Hill, T. D., and Angel, R. J. (2005). Neighborhood disorder, psychological distress, and heavy drinking. *Social Science and Medicine, 61*, 965–75.

Hladik, F., and Hope, T. J. (2009). HIV infection in the genital mucosa of women. *Current HIV/AIDS Reports, 6(1)*, 20–28.

Hogan, M. F. (2002). Chairman's cover letter for the interim report to President George W. Bush. May 29. President's New Freedom Commission on Mental Health, Washington, DC.

Holtgrave, D. R., Qualls, N. L., Curran, J. W., Valdiserri, R. O., Guinan, M. E., and Parra, W. C. (1995). An overview of the effectiveness and efficacy of HIV prevention programs. *Public Health Reports, 10(2)*, 134–46.

Horowitz, R. (1983). *Honor and the American dream: Culture and identity in a Chicano community.* New Brunswick, NJ: Rutgers University Press.

Horwitz, A. V., Reinhard, S. C., and Howell-White, S. (1996). Caregiving as reciprocal exchange in families with seriously mentally ill members. *Journal of Health and Social Behavior, 37*, 149–62.

Hough, R. L., Tarke, H., Renker, V., Shields, P., and Glatstein, J. (1996). Recruitment and retention of homeless mentally ill participants in research. *Journal of Consulting and Clinical Psychology, 64(5)*, 881–91.

Hudson, C. G. (2005). Socioeconomic status and mental illness: Tests of the social causation and selection hypotheses. *American Journal of Orthopsychiatry, 75(1)*, 3–18.

Hulme, P. A. (2004). Theoretical perspectives on the health problems of adults who experienced childhood sexual abuse. *Issues in Mental Health Nursing, 25*, 339–61.

Hutchings, P., and Dutton, M. (1993). Sexual assault history in a community mental health center clinic population. *Community Mental Health Journal, 29*, 59–63.

Jacobson, J. O., Robinson, P., and Bluthenthal, R. N. (2007). A multilevel decomposition approach to estimate the role of program location and neighborhood disadvantage in racial disparities in alcohol treatment completion. *Social Science and Medicine, 64*, 462–76.

Jaffee, S. R., and Price, T. S. (2007). Gene-environment correlations: A review of the evidence and implications for prevention of mental illness. *Molecular Psychiatry, 12*, 432–42.

Janoff-Bulman, R. (1992). *Shattered assumptions: Toward a new psychology of trauma.* New York: Free Press.

Janz, N. K., and Becker, M. H. (1984). The health belief model: A decade later. *Health Education Quarterly, 11*, 1–47.

Jenkins, J. H. (1988). Ethnopsychiatric interpretations of schizophrenic illness: The problem of *nervios* within Mexican-American families. *Culture, Medicine, and Psychiatry, 12*, 301–29.

Johnson-Masotti, A. P., Weinhardt, L. S., Pinkerton, S. D., and Otto-Salaj, L. L. (2003). Efficacy and cost-effectiveness of the first generation of HIV prevention interventions for people with severe and persistent mental illness. *Journal of Mental Health Policy Economics, 6(1)*, 23–35.

Jones, E. E., Farina, A., Hastorf, A., Markus, H., Millar, D. S., and Scott, R. A. (1984). *Social stigma: The psychology of marked relationships*. New York: W. H. Freeman.

Kaiser Permanente National Diversity Council. (2001). *A provider's handbook on culturally competent care: Latino population.* Oakland, CA: Kaiser Permanente National Diversity Council.

Kalichman, S. C., Belcher, L., Cherry, C., and Williams, E. A. (1997). Primary prevention of sexually transmitted infections: Transferring behavioral research technology to community programs. *Journal of Primary Prevention, 18(2)*, 149–72.

Kalichman, S. C., Heckman, T. G., and Kelly, J. A. (1996). Sensation seeking as an explanation for the association between substance use and HIV-related risky sexual behavior. *Archives of Sexual Behavior, 25*, 141–54.

Kalichman, S. C., Kelly, J. A., Johnson, J. R., and Bulton, M. (1994). Factors associated with risk for HIV infection among chronically mentally ill adults. *American Journal of Psychiatry, 151*, 221–27.

Kantor, G. K., Jasinski, J. L., and Aldarondo, E. (1994). Sociocultural status and incidence of marital violence in Hispanic families. *Violence and Victims, 9(3)*, 207–22.

Kapur, S., and Remington, G. (2000). Atypical antipsychotics. *British Medical Journal, 321*, 1360–61.

Katz, R. C., Watts, C., and Santman, J. (1994). AIDS knowledge and high risk behaviors in the chronically mentally ill. *Community Mental Health Journal, 30*, 395–402.

Kelly, B. D. (2006). The power gap: Freedom, power, and mental illness. *Social Science and Medicine, 63*, 2118–28.

Kelly, B. D. (2005). Structural violence and schizophrenia. *Social Science and Medicine, 61*, 721–30.

Kelly, J. A. (1997). HIV risk reduction interventions for persons with severe mental illness. *Clinical Psychology Review, 17(3)*, 293–309.

Kelly, J. A., Murphy, D. A., Bahr, G. R., Brasfield, T. L., Davis, D. R., Hauth, H. C., Morgan, M. G., Stevenson, L. Y., and Eilers, M. K. (1992). AIDS/HIV risk behavior among the chronically mentally ill. *American Journal of Psychiatry, 149*, 886–89.

Kelly, J. A., Murphy, D. A., Sikkema, K. J., Somlai, A. M., Mulry, G. W., Fernandez, M. I., Miller, J. G., and Stevenson, L. Y. (1995). Predictors of high and low levels of HIV risk behavior among adults with chronic mental illness. *Psychiatric Services, 46*, 813–18.

Kendrick, T. (1999). The newer, "atypical" antipsychotic drugs—their development and current therapeutic use. *British Journal of General Practice, 49*, 745–49.

Kenny, D. A., and Acitelli, L. K. (2001). Accuracy and bias in the perception of the partner in close relationships. *Journal of Personality and Social Psychology, 80*, 434–48.

Kessler, R. C., McGonagle, K. A., Zhao, S., Nelson, C. B., Hughes, M., Eshleman, S., Wittchen, H. U., and Kendler, K. S. (1994). Lifetime and 12-month prevalence of DSM-III-R psychiatric disorders in the United States. *Archives of General Psychiatry, 51*, 8–19.

Kety, S. S., Rosenthal, D., Wender, P. H., Schulsinger, F., and Jacobsen, B. (1976). Mental illness in the biological and adoptive families of adopted individuals who have become schizophrenic. *Behavior Genetics, 6(3)*, 219–25.

Khantzian, E. J. (1997). The self-medication hypothesis of substance use disorders: A reconsideration and recent applications. *Harvard Review of Psychiatry, 4*, 231–44.

Kilcommons, A. M., and Morrison, A. P. (2005). Relationships between trauma and psychosis: An exploration of cognitive and dissociative factors. *Acta Psychiatrica Scandinavica, 112*, 351–59.

Kim, A., Galanter, M., Castaneda, R., Lifshutz, H., and Franco, H. (1992). Crack cocaine use and sexual behavior among psychiatric inpatients. *American Journal of Drug and Alcohol Abuse, 18*, 235–46.

King, T. E., Wheeler, M. B., Bindman, A. B., Fernandez, A., Grumbach, K., Schillinger, D., and Villela, T. J. (2007). *Medical management of vulnerable and underserved patients: Principles, practice, and populations.* New York: McGraw Hill.

Kinzl, J., and Biebl, W. (1991). Sexual abuse of girls: Aspects of the genesis of mental disorders and therapeutic implications. *Acta Psychiatrica Scandinavica, 83*, 427–31.

Kisiel, C. L., and Lyons, J. S. (2001). Dissociation as a mediator of psychopathology among sexually abused children and adolescents. *American Journal of Psychiatry, 158(7)*, 1034–39.

Klehr, K. B., Cohler, B. J., and Musick, J. S. (1983). Character and behavior in the mentally ill and well mother. *Infant Mental Health Journal, 4*, 250–70.

Klein, H., and Chao, B. (1995). Sexual abuse during childhood and adolescence as predictors of HIV-related sexual risk during adulthood among female sexual partners of injection drug users. *Violence against Women, 1(1)*, 55–76.

Kleinman, A. (1996). How is culture important for DSM-IV? In J. Mezzich, A. Kleinman, H. Fabrega, and D. Parron (Eds.). *Culture and psychiatric diagnosis: A DSM-IV perspective* (pp. 15–26). Washington, DC: American Psychiatric Press.

Knox, M. D., Boaz, T. L., Friedrich, M. A., and Dow, M. D. (1994). HIV risk factors for persons with severe mental illness. *Community Mental Health Journal, 30*, 551–63.

Knudsen, P., and Vilmar, T. (1984). Cannabis and neuroleptic agents in schizophrenia. *Acta Psychiatrica Scandinavica, 69*, 162–74.

Koegel, P., Sullivan, G., Burnam, A., Morton, S. C., and Wenzel, S. (1999). Utilization of mental health and substance abuse services among homeless adults in Los Angeles. *Medical Care, 37*, 306–17.

Koob, G. F., and Le Moal, M. (1997). Drug abuse: Hedonic homeostatic dysregulation. *Science, 278*, 52–58.

Koss, M. P. (1993). Rape: Scope, impact, interventions, and public policy responses. *American Psychologist, 48*, 1062–69.

Kroll, J., and Sheehan, W. (1989). Religious beliefs and practices among 52 psychiatric inpatients in Minnesota. *American Journal of Psychiatry, 146*, 67–72.

Kruglanski, A. W., and Webster, D. M. (1996). Motivated closing of the mind: "Seizing" and "freezing." *Psychological Review, 103(2)*, 263–83.

Kushel, M. B., Evans, J. L., Perry, S., Robertson, M. J., and Moss, A. R. (2003). No door to lock: Victimization among homeless and marginally housed persons. *Archives of Internal Medicine, 163*, 2492–99.

Laing, R. D. (1960). *The divided self: An existential study in sanity and madness.* Harmondsworth, UK: Penguin.

Laing, R. D. (1961). *Self and others.* Harmondsworth, UK: Penguin.

Lamb, H. R., and Lamb, D. M. (1990). Factors contributing to homelessness among the chronically and severely mentally ill. *Hospital and Community Psychiatry, 41(3)*, 301–5.

Lapalme, M., Hodgins, S., and LaRoche, C. (1997). Children of parents with bipolar disorder: A metaanalysis of risk for mental disorders. *Canadian Journal of Psychiatry, 42*, 623–31.

Lapp, M. (1986). *The migration division of Puerto Rico and Puerto Ricans living in New York City, 1948–1969.* New York: New York Historical Society.

Larsson, B., Knuttson-Medin, L., Sundelin, C., and Trost von Werder, A. C. (2000). Social competence and emotional/behavioural problems in children of psychiatric inpatients. *European Child and Adolescent Psychiatry, 9*, 122–28.

Latkin, C. A., and Curry, A. D. (2003). Stressful neighborhoods and depression: A prospective study of the impact of neighborhood disorder. *Journal of Health and Social Behavior, 44*, 34–44.

Laumann, E. O., Gagnon, J. H., Michael, R. T., and Michael, S. (1994). *The social organization of sexuality*. Chicago: University of Chicago Press.

Launer, J. (1999). A narrative approach to mental health in general practice. *British Medical Journal, 318*, 117–19.

Lawthers, A. G., Pransky, G. S., Peterson, L. E., and Himmelstein, J. H. (2003). Rethinking quality in the context of persons with disability. *International Journal for Quality in Health Care, 15(4)*, 287–99.

Leaf, P. J., Bruce, M. L., and Tischler, G. L. (1986). The differential effect of attitudes on the use of mental health services. *Social Psychiatry, 21*, 187–92.

Leaf, P. J., Bruce, M. L., Tischler, G. L., and Holzer, C. E. (1987). The relationship between demographic factors and attitudes toward mental health services. *Journal of Community Psychology, 15*, 275–84.

Lechner, M. E., Vogel, M. E., Garcia-Shelton, L. M., Leichter, J. L., and Steibel, K. R. (1993). Self-reported medical problems of adult female survivors of childhood sexual abuse. *Journal of Family Practice, 36*, 633–38.

Lederman, S. A., and Sierra, D. (1994). Characteristics of childbearing Hispanic women in New York City. In G. Lamberty and C. Garcia Coll (Eds.). *Puerto Rican women and children: Issues in health, growth, and development* (pp. 85–102). New York: Plenum.

Lehman, A. F. (1995). Vocational rehabilitation in schizophrenia. *Schizophrenia Bulletin, 21*, 645–56.

Lehman, A. F., Dixon, L., Hoch, J. S., Deforge, B., Kernan, E., and Frank, R. (1999). Cost-effectiveness of assertive community treatment for homeless persons with severe mental illness. *British Journal of Psychiatry, 174*, 346–52.

Lehman, A. F., Goldberg, R., Dixon, L. B., McNary, S., Postrado, L., Hackman, A., and McDonnell, K. (2002). Improving employment outcomes for persons with severe mental illness. *Archives of General Psychiatry, 59*, 165–72.

Lemert, E. M. (1951). *Social pathology*. New York: McGraw-Hill.

Lemp, G., Jones, M., Kellogg, T., Nieri, G., Anderson, L., Withum, D., and Katz, M. (1995). HIV seroprevalence and risk behaviors among lesbians and bisexual women in San Francisco and Berkeley, California. *American Journal of Public Health, 85 (11)*, 1549–52.

Lesbian AIDS Project. (1994). *Results of the Lesbian AIDS Project's Women's Sex Survey: Final report.* New York: Lesbian AIDS Project/Gay Men's Health Crisis.

Leucht, S., Pitschel-Walz, G., Abraham, D., and Kissling, W. (1999). Efficacy and extrapyramidal side-effects of the new antipsychotics olanzapine, quetiapine, risperidone, and sertindole compared to conventional antipsychotics and placebo: A meta-analysis of randomized controlled trials. *Schizophrenia Research, 35*, 51–68.

Levendosky, A. A., and Graham-Bermann, S. A. (2001). Parenting in battered women: The effects of domestic violence on women and their children. *Journal of Family Violence, 16(2)*, 171–92.

Levitan, R. D., Rector, N. A., Sheldon, T., and Goering, P. (2003). Childhood adversities associated with major depression and/or anxiety disorders in a community sample of Ontario: Issues of co-morbidity and specificity. *Depression and Anxiety, 17*, 34–42.

Lewis-Fernández, R. (1996). Cultural formulation of psychiatric diagnosis. *Culture, Medicine, and Psychiatry, 20*, 155–63.

Lieb, R., Isensee, B., Hofler, M., Pfister, H., and Wittchen, H. (2002). Parental major depression and the risk of depression and other mental disorders in offspring: A prospective-longitudinal community study. *Archives of General Psychiatry, 59(4)*, 365–74.

Liebowitz, M. R., Quitkin, F. M., Stewart, J. W., McGrath, P. J., Harrison, W., Rabkin, J. G., Tricamo, E., Markowitz, J. S., and Klein, D. F. (1994). Psychopharmacological validation of atypical depression. *Journal of Clinical Psychiatry, 45(7)*, 22–25.

Lillie-Blanton, M., Martinez, R. M., Taylor, A. K., and Robinson, R. M. (1993). Latina and African American women: Continuing disparities in health. *International Journal of Health Services, 23(3)*, 555–84.

Lin, K.-M. (2001). Biological differences in depression and anxiety across races and groups. *Journal of Clinical Psychiatry, 62 (Suppl. 13)*, 13–19; discussion 20–21.

Lindgren, K. N., and Coursey, R. D. (1995). Spirituality and mental illness: A two-part study. *Psychosocial Rehabilitation Journal, 18(3)*, 93–111.

Link, B. G. (1987). Understanding labeling effects in the area of mental disorders: An assessment of the effects of expectations of rejection. *American Sociological Review, 52*, 96–112.

Link, B. G. (1982). Mental patient status, work, and income: An examination of the effects of a psychiatric label. *American Sociological Review, 47*, 202–15.

Link, B. G., Cullen, F. T., Frank, J., and Wozniak, J. F. (1987). The social rejection of former mental patients: Understanding why labels matter. *American Journal of Sociology, 92*, 1461–1500.

Link, B. G., Cullen, F. T., Struening, E., Shrout, P., and Dohrenwend, B. P. (1989). A modified labeling theory approach to mental disorders: An empirical assessment. *American Sociological Review, 54*, 400–423.

Link, B. G., Mirotznik, J., and Cullen, F. T. (1991). The effectiveness of stigma coping orientations: Can negative consequences of mental illness labeling be avoided? *Journal of Health and Social Behavior, 32(3)*, 302–20.

Link, B. G., and Phelan, J. C. (2001). Conceptualizing stigma. *Annual Review of Sociology, 27*, 363–85.

Link, B. G., Phelan, J. C., Bresnahan, M., Stueve, A., and Pescosolido, B. A. (1999). Public conceptions of mental illness: Labels, causes, dangerousness, and social distance. *American Journal of Public Health, 89(9)*, 1328–33.

Longshore, D., Stein, J. A., and Anglin, M. D. (1996). Ethnic differences in the psychosocial antecedents of needle/syringe disinfection. *Drug and Alcohol Dependence, 42*, 183–96.

Lopez, S. (1989). Patient variable biases in clinical judgment: Conceptual overview and methodological considerations. *Psychology Bulletin, 106*, 184–203.

Lorei, T. W. (1967). Prediction of community stay and employment for released patients. *Journal of Consulting Psychology, 31*, 349–57.

Loue, S. (2001). *Intimate partner violence.* New York: Kluwer Academic/Plenum.

Loue, S., Cooper, M., and Fiedler, J. (2003a). HIV Knowledge among a sample of Puerto Rican and Mexican men and women. *Journal of Immigrant Health, 5*, 59–66.

Loue, S., Cooper, M., and Fiedler, J. (2003b). HIV Risk among a sample of Mexican and Puerto Rican men and women. *Journal of Health Care for the Poor and Underserved, 14*, 550–65.

Loue, S., Cooper, M., Traore, F., and Fiedler, J. (2004). Locus of control and HIV risk among a sample of Mexican and Puerto Rican women. *Journal of Immigrant Health, 6(4)*, 155–65.

Loue, S., and Mendez, N. (2006). "I don't know who I am": Severely mentally ill Latina WSW navigating differentness. *Journal of Lesbian Studies, 10(1–2)*, 249–66.

Loue, S., and Sajatovic, M. (2006).

Spirituality, coping, and HIV risk and prevention in a sample of severely mentally ill Puerto Rican women. *Journal of Urban Health, 83(6)*, 1168–82.

Low, S. (1981). The meaning of *nervios*: A sociocultural analysis of symptom presentation in San Jose, Costa Rica. *Culture, Medicine, and Psychiatry, 5*, 25–47.

Lown, E. A., and Vega, W. A. (2001). Alcohol abuse or dependence among Mexican American women who report violence. *Alcoholism: Clinical and Experimental Research, 25(10)*, 1479–86.

Lugo Steidel, A. G., and Contreras, J. M. (2003). A new familism scale for use with Latino populations. *Hispanic Journal of Behavioral Sciences, 25(3)*, 312–30.

Lukianowicz, N. (1972). Incest. *British Journal of Psychiatry, 120*, 301–13.

Lundin, R. (1997). Mental illness and spirituality: A personal view. *Journal of the California Alliance for the Mentally Ill, 8*, 46–48.

Lysaker, P. H., Davis, L. W., Warman, D. M., Strasburger, A., and Beattie, N. (2007). Stigma, social function and symptoms in schizophrenia and schizoaffective disorder: Associations across 6 months. *Psychiatry Research, 149*, 89–95.

Macmillan, H. L., Fleming, J. E., Streiner, D. L., Lin, E., Boyle, M. H., Jamieson, E., et al. (2001). Childhood abuse and lifetime psychopathology in a community sample. *American Journal of Psychiatry, 158*, 1878–83.

Maisch, H. (1972). *Incest*. Trans. C. Bearne. New York: Stein and Day.

Maj, M., Akiskal, H. S., Lopez-Ibor, J. J., and Sartorius, N. (Eds.) (2002). *Bipolar disorder*. West Sussex, UK: John Wiley and Sons.

Maldonado, E. (1979). Contract labor and the origins of Puerto Rican communities in the United States. *International Migration Review, 13*, 103–21.

Malow, R., Dévieux, J. G., Martinez, L., Peipman, F., Lucenko, B. A., and Kalichman, S. C. (2006). History of traumatic abuse and HIV risk behaviors in severely mentally ill substance abusing adults. *Journal of Family Violence, 21(2)*, 127–35.

Marchevsky, A., and Theoharis, J. (2006). *Not working: Latina immigrants, low-wage jobs, and the failure of welfare reform*. New York: New York University Press.

Marcos, L. R. (1976). Bilinguals in psychotherapy: Language as an emotional barrier. *American Journal of Psychotherapy, 30*, 552–59.

Marcos, L. R., Alpert, M., Urcuyo, L., and Kesselman, M. (1973). The effect of interview language in the evaluation of psychopathology in Spanish American schizophrenic patients. *American Journal of Psychiatry, 130*, 549–53.

Marcos, L. R., and Urcuyo, L. (1979). Dynamic psychotherapy with the bilingual patient. *American Journal of Psychotherapy, 33*, 331–38.

Marcotte, E., Wilcox-Gök, V., and Redmon, D. P. (2000). The labor market effects of mental illness: The case of affective disorders. In D. Salkever (Ed.). *The economics of disability* (pp. 123–31). Greenwich, CT: JAI Press.

Marín, B. V. (2003). HIV prevention in the Hispanic community: Sex, culture, and empowerment. *Journal of Transcultural Nursing, 14*, 186–92.

Marín, B. V. (1996). Cultural issues in HIV prevention for Latinos: Should we try to change gender roles? In S. Oskamp and S. C. Thompson (Eds.). *Understanding and preventing HIV risk behavior: Safer sex and drug use* (pp. 157–76). Newbury Park, CA: Sage.

Marín, B. V., Gómez, C. A., Tschann, J. M., and Gregorich, S. E. (1997). Condom use in unmarried Latino men: A test of cultural constructs. *Health Psychology, 16(5)*, 458–67.

Marín, G. (1989). AIDS prevention among Hispanics: Needs, risk behaviors, and cultural values. *Public Health Reports, 104(5)*, 411–15.

Marín, G., and Gamba, R. J. (1996). A

new measurement of acculturation for Hispanics: The Bidimensional Acculturation Scale for Hispanics (BAS). *Hispanic Journal of Behavioral Sciences, 18*, 297–316.

Marín, G., and Marín, B. V. (1991). *Research with Hispanic populations*. Newbury Park, CA: Sage.

Marin, H., and Escobar, J. I. (2001). Special issues in the psychopharmacological management of U.S. Hispanics. *Psychopharmacology Bulletin, 35*, 197–212.

Marks, G., and Miller, N. (1987). Ten years of research on the false consensus effect: An empirical and theoretical review. *Psychological Bulletin, 102*, 72–90.

Markus, H., and Cross. S. (1990). The interpersonal self. In L. Pervin (Ed.). *Handbook of personality: Theory and research* (pp. 576–608). New York: Guilford Press.

Marshall, T., Solomon, P., Steber, S.-A., and Mannion, E. (2003). Provider and family beliefs regarding the causes of severe mental illness. *Psychiatric Quarterly, 74(3)*, 223–36.

Martinez, R., and Dukes, R. (1991). Ethnic and gender differences in self-esteem. *Youth and Society, 22*, 318–38.

Marwaha, S., and Johnson, J. (2004). Schizophrenia and employment: A review. *Social Psychiatry and Psychiatric Epidemiology, 39*, 337–49.

Maslow, A. H. (1970). *Motivation and personality*, 2nd ed. New York: Harper and Row.

Mathews, C. A., Glidden, D., Murray, S., Forster, P., and Hargreaves, W. A. (2002). The effect on treatment outcomes of assigning patients to ethnically focused inpatient psychiatric units. *Psychiatric Services, 53(7)*, 830–35.

Mattson, S., and Rodriguez, E. (1999). Battering in pregnant Latinas. *Issues in Mental Health Nursing, 20*, 405–22.

Maxwell, B., and Jacobson, M. (1989). *Marketing disease to Hispanics: The selling of alcohol, tobacco, and junk foods.* Washington, DC: Center for Science in the Public Interest.

McBride, C. A. (1998). The discounting principle and attitudes towards victims of HIV infection. *Journal of Applied Social Psychology, 28(7)*, 595–608.

McCauley, J., Kern, D. E., Kolodner, K., Dill, L., Schroeder, A. F., DeChant, H. K., Ryden, J., Derogatis, L. R., and Bass, E. B. (1997). Clinical characteristics of women with a history of childhood abuse. *Journal of the American Medical Association, 277*, 1362–68.

McClure, S. M., Laibson, D. I., Loewenstein, G., and Cohen, J. D. (2004). Separate neural systems value immediate and delayed monetary rewards. *Science, 306(5695)*, 503–7.

McCord, W., and McCord, J. (1960). *Origins of alcoholism*. Stanford, CA: Stanford University Press.

McCrae, J. S., Chapman, M. V., and Christ, S. L. (2006). Profile of children investigated for sexual abuse: Association with psychopathology symptoms and services. *American Journal of Orthopsychiatry, 76(4)*, 468–81.

McDermott, B. E., Sautter, F. J., Jr., Winstead, D. K., and Quirk, T. (1994). Diagnosis, health beliefs, and risk of HIV infection in psychiatric patients. *Hospital and Community Psychiatry, 45*, 580–85.

McFarlane, J., and Parker, B. (1995). *Abuse during pregnancy: A protocol for prevention and intervention*. White Plains, NY: March of Dimes Birth Defects Foundation.

McFarlane, J., Soeken, K., Reel, S., Parker, B., and Silva, C. (1997). Resource use by abused women following an intervention program: Associated severity of abuse and reports of abuse ending. *Public Health Nursing, 14(4)*, 244–50.

McFarlane, J., Wiist, W., and Watson, M. (1998a). Characteristics of sexual abuse against pregnant Hispanic women by their male intimates. *Journal of Women's Health, 7(6)*, 739–45.

McFarlane, J., Wiist, W., and Watson, M. (1998b). Predicting physical abuse against pregnant Hispanic women.

American Journal of Preventive Medicine, 15(2), 134–38.

McGurk, S. R., and Mueser, K. T. (2004). Cognitive functioning, symptoms, and work in supported employment: A review and heuristic model. *Schizophrenia Research, 70*, 147–73.

McKenzie, K. (2002). Understanding racism in mental health. In K. Bui (Ed.). *Racism and mental health: Prejudice and suffering* (pp. 83–99). London: Jessica Kingsley.

McKinnon, K., Cournos, F., Sugden, R., Guido, J. R., and Herman, R. (1996). The relative contributions of psychiatric symptoms and AIDS knowledge to HIV risk behaviors among people with severe mental illness. *Journal of Clinical Psychiatry, 57*, 506–13.

McQuillan, G. M., Khare, M., Karon, J. M., Schable, C. A., and Vlahov, D. (1997). Update on the seroepidemiology of human immunodeficiency virus in the United States household population: NHANES III, 1988–1994. *Journal of Acquired Immune Deficiency Syndromes and Human Retrovirology, 4*, 355–60.

Mead, G. H. (1934). *Mind, self, and society.* Chicago: University of Chicago Press.

Meade, C. S., Kershaw, T. S., Hansen, N. B., and Sikkema, K. J. (2009). Long-term correlates of childhood abuse among adults with severe mental illness: Adult victimization, substance abuse, and HIV sexual risk behavior. *AIDS Behavior, 13*, 207–16.

Meade, C. S., and Sikkema, K. J. (2005). Voluntary HIV testing among adults with severe mental illness: Frequency and associated factors. *AIDS Behavior, 9(4)*, 465–73.

Medlicott, R. (1967). Parent-child incest. *Australian and New Zealand Journal of Psychiatry, 1*, 180–87.

Mehlman, R. D. (1961). The Puerto Rican syndrome. *American Journal of Psychiatry, 118*, 328–32.

Metts, S., and Spitzberg, B. H. (1996). Sexual communication in interpersonal contexts: A script-based approach. In B. Burleson (Ed.). *Communication Yearbook*, vol. 19 (pp. 49–91). Mahwah, NJ: Erlbaum.

Meyer, I., Cournos, F., Empfield, M., Schrage, H., Silver, M., Rubin, M., and Weinstock, A. (1993). HIV seroprevalence and clinical characteristics of the mentally ill homeless. *Journal of Social Distress and the Homeless, 2*, 103–16.

Meyer, I., McKinnon, K., Cournos, F., Empfield, M., Bavlis, S., Engel, D., and Weinstock, A. (1993). HIV seroprevalence among long-stay psychiatric patients. *Hospital and Community Psychiatry, 44*, 282–84.

Mikawa, J. K., Morones, P. A., Gomez, A., Case, H. L., Olsen, D., and Gonzales-Huss, M. J. (1992). Cultural practices of Hispanics: Implications for the prevention of AIDS. *Hispanic Journal of Behavioral Sciences, 14(4)*, 421–33.

Millar, A. B., and Gruenewald, P. J. (1997). Use of spatial models for community program evaluation of changes in alcohol outlet distribution. *Addiction, 92*, 273–84.

Miller, B. A, Downs, W. R., and Gondoli, D. M. (1989). Spousal violence among alcoholic women as compared to a random household sample of women. *Journal of Studies on Alcohol, 50*, 533–40.

Miller, B. A, Downs, W. R., and Testa, M. (1993). Interrelationships between victimization experiences and women's alcohol use. *Journal of Studies on Alcohol, 11*, 109–17.

Miller, J. E., Guarnaccia, P. J., and Fasina, A. (2002). AIDS knowledge among Latinos: The roles of language, culture, and socioeconomic status. *Journal of Immigrant Health, 4(2)*, 63–72.

Miller, K. S., Clark, L. F., and Moore, J. S. (1997). Sexual initiation with older male partners and subsequent HIV risk behavior among female adolescents. *Family Planning Perspectives, 29*, 212–14.

Miller, M. (1999). A model to explain the relationship between sexual abuse and

HIV risk among women. *AIDS Care, 11(1)*, 3–20.

Miller, M., and Paone, D. (1998). Social network characteristics as mediators in the relationship between sexual abuse and HIV risk. *Social Science and Medicine, 47(6)*, 765–77.

Miller, R. J., and Finnerty, M. (1996). Sexuality, pregnancy, and childrearing among women with schizophrenia-spectrum disorders. *Psychiatric Services, 47(5)*, 502–6.

Mills, C. W., Senior, C., and Goldsen, R. (1950). *The Puerto Rican journey: New York's newest migrants*. New York: Harper Press.

Minsky, S., Vega, W., Miskimen, T., Gara, M., and Escobar, J. (2003). Diagnostic patterns in Latino, African American, and European American psychiatric patients. *Archives of General Psychiatry, 60*, 637–44.

Miranda, J., and Cooper, L. A. (2004). Disparities in care for depression among primary care patients. *Journal of General Internal Medicine, 19*, 120–26.

Miranda, J., Lawson, W., Escobar, J., and NIMH Affective Disorders Workgroup. (2002). Ethnic minorities. *Mental Health Services Research, 4(4)*, 231–37.

Mirandé, A. (1988). Que gacho es ser macho: It's a drag to be a macho man. *Aztlan, 17*, 63–69.

Mishra, S. I., Sanudo, F., and Conner, R. F. (2004). Collaborative research toward HIV prevention among migrant farmworkers. In B. P. Bowser, S. I. Mishra, C. J. Reback, and G. F. Lemp (Eds.). *Preventing AIDS: Community-science collaborations* (pp. 69–95). New York: Haworth Press.

Mitchell, L., and Romans, S. (2002). Spiritual beliefs in bipolar affective disorder: Their relevance for illness management. *Journal of Affective Disorders, 75*, 247–57.

Mizio, E. (1977). Commentary: Additional thoughts are presented regarding the needs of, knowledge of, and sensitivity to cultural factors in relation to Puerto Rican clients. *Social Casework*, Oct., 471.

Molnar, B. E., Buka, S. L., and Kessler, R. C. (2001). Child sexual abuse and subsequent psychopathology: Results from the National Comorbidity Survey. *American Journal of Public Health, 91(5)*, 753–60.

Moore, A. J., Williams, J. D., and Qualls, W. J. (1996). Target marketing of tobacco and alcohol-related products to ethnic minority groups in the United States. *Ethnicity and Disease, 6*, 83–98.

Morrison, A. P. (2001). The interpretation of intrusions in psychosis: An integrative cognitive approach to hallucinations and delusions. *Behavioral Cognitive Psychotherapy, 29*, 257–76.

Morrison, R. L., and Bellack, A. S. (1987). Social functioning in schizophrenia patients: Clinical and research issues. *Schizophrenia Bulletin, 13*, 715–25.

Morrissey, J. P, and Dennis, D. L. (1990). *Homelessness and mental illness: Toward the next generation of research studies.* Rockville, MD: National Institute of Mental Health.

Morrow, K. M., and Allsworth, J. E. (2000). Sexual risk in lesbians and bisexual women. *Journal of the Gay and Lesbian Medical Association, 4(4)*, 159–65.

Morton, M. J. (2000). Institutionalizing inequalities: Black children and child welfare in Cleveland, 1859–1998. *Journal of Social History, 34(1)*, 141–62.

Mowbray, C. T., Oyserman, D., and Ross, S. (1995). Parenting and the significance of children for women with a serious mental illness. *Journal of Mental Health Administration, 22*, 189–200.

Muehlenhard, C. L., Highby, B. J., Lee, R. S., Bryan, T. S., and Dodrill, W. A. (1998). The sexual revictimization of women and men sexually abused as children: A review of the literature. *Annual Review of Sex Research, 9*, 177–223.

Muenzenmaier, K., Meyer, I., Struening, E., and Ferber, J. (1993). Childhood abuse and neglect among women outpatients with chronic mental illness. *Hospital and Community Psychiatry, 44*, 666–70.

Mueser, K. T., Bond, G. R., Drake, R. E., and Resnick, S. (1998). Model of community care for severe mental illness: A review of research on case management. *Schizophrenia Bulletin, 24*, 37–74.

Mueser, K. T., Goodman, L. A., Trumbetta, S. L., Rosenberg, S. D., Osher, F. C., Vidaver, R., et al. (1998). Trauma and posttraumatic stress disorder in severe mental illness. *Journal of Consulting and Clinical Psychology, 66*, 493–99.

Mueser, K. T., Rosenberg, S. D., Goodman, L. A., and Trumbetta, S. L. (2002). Trauma, PTSD, and the course of severe mental illness: An interactive model. *Schizophrenia Research, 53*, 123–43.

Mueser, K. T., Salyers, M. P., Rosenberg, S. D., Ford, J. D., Fox, L., and Carty, P. (2001). Psychometric evaluation of trauma and posttraumatic stress disorder assessments in persons with severe mental illness. *Psychological Assessments, 13*, 110–17.

Mulder, R. T., Beautrais, A. L., Joyce, P. R., and Fergusson, D. M. (1998). Relationship between dissociation, childhood sexual abuse, childhood physical abuse, and mental illness in a general population sample. *American Journal of Psychiatry, 155(6)*, 806–11.

Muntaner, C., Pulver, A. E., McGrath, J., and Eaton, W. W. (1993). Work environment and schizophrenia: An extension of the arousal hypothesis to occupational self-selection. *Social Psychiatry and Psychiatric Epidemiology, 28*, 231–38.

Murray, S., Holmes, J. G., and Griffin, D. W. (1996). The benefits of positive illusions: Idealization and the construction of satisfaction in close relationships. *Journal of Personality and Social Psychology, 70*, 79–98.

Nagoshi, C. T., Wilson, J. R., and Rodriguez, L. A. (1991). Impulsivity, sensation seeking, and behavioral and emotional responses to alcohol. *Alcoholism: Clinical and Experimental Research, 15*, 661–67.

National Drug Intelligence Center. (2004). *Drug abuse and mental illness: Fast facts.* Washington, DC: U.S. Department of Justice.

National Institute on Drug Abuse. (2008). *MDMA (ecstasy).* Rockville, MD: U.S. Department of Health and Human Services, August.

Neff, J. A., Holamon, B., and Schluter, T. D. (1995). Spousal violence among Anglos, Blacks, and Mexican Americans: The role of demographic variables, psychosocial predictors, and alcohol consumption. *Journal of Family Violence, 10*, 1–21.

Nicolosi, A., Leite, M. L. C., Musicco, M., Arici, C., Gavazzeni, G., and Lazzarin, A. (1994). The efficiency of male-to-female and female-to-male sexual transmission of the human immunodeficiency virus: A study of 730 stable couples. *Epidemiology, 5(6)*, 570–75.

NIMH Multisite HIV Prevention Trial Group. (2001). A test of factors mediating the relationship between unwanted sexual activity during childhood and risky sexual practices among women enrolled in the NIMH Multisite HIV Prevention Trial. *Women and Health, 33(1–2)*, 163–80.

Niquette, N., Candisky, C., and Johnson, A. (2008). Ax taken to state jobs; Strickland will cut spending; up to 2,700 jobs to cover shortfall. *Columbus Dispatch*, Feb. 1. Retrieved April 24, 2009, from *www.mentalhealthadvocacy.org/News_Strickland%20will%20cut%spending.pdf.*

Noland, C. M. (2006). Listen to the sound of silence: Gender roles and communication about sex in Puerto Rico. *Sex Roles, 55*, 283–94.

Nomura, Y., Wickramaratne, P. J., Warner, V., Mufson, L., and Weissman, M. M. (2002). Family discord, parental depression, and psychopathology in offspring: Ten-year follow-up. *Journal of the American Academy of Child and Adolescent Psychiatry, 41*, 402–9.

Norland, C. M. (2006). Listening to the sound of silence: Gender roles and communication about sex in Puerto Rico. *Sex Roles, 55*, 283–94.

North, C. S., and Smith, E. M. (1993). A systematic study of mental health services utilization by homeless men and women. *Social Psychiatry and Psychiatric Epidemiology, 28*, 77–83.

Norton, W. E., Amico, K. R., Cornman, D. H., Fisher, W. A., and Fisher, J. D. (2009). An agenda for advancing the science of implementation of evidence-based HIV prevention interventions. *AIDS Behavior* (e-pub ahead of print).

Nyamathi, A. M., Flaskerud, J., Bennett, C., Leake, B., and Lewis, C. (1994). Evaluation of two AIDS programs for impoverished Latina women. *AIDS Education and Prevention, 6*, 296–309.

Oberg, K. (1960). Culture shock: Adjustment to new cultural environments. *Practical Anthropology, 7*, 177–82.

Oberg, K. (1954). Culture shock. Bobbs-Merrill Reprint Series in the Social Sciences, A-329. Indianapolis, IN: Bobbs-Merrill. Retrieved March 7, 2009, from *www.smcm.edu/academics/internationaled/Pdf/cultureshockarticle.pdf.*

Office of Applied Statistics, Substance Abuse and Mental Health Services Administration. (2005). Substance use during pregnancy: 2002 and 2003 update. *National Survey on Drug Use and Health (NSDUH) Report.* Retrieved January 2008 from *www.oas.samhsa.gov.*

Ohio State University. (1991). *The Hispanic action plan.* Columbus, OH: Ohio State University. Retrieved May 22, 2009, from *quepasa.osu.edu/actionplan.pdf.*

Onwuegbuzie, A. J., and Teddlie, C. (2003). A framework for analyzing data in mixed methods research. In A. Tashakkori and C. Teddlie (Eds.). *Handbook of mixed methods in social and behavioral research* (pp. 351–83). Thousand Oaks, CA: Sage.

Opolka, J. L., Rascati, K. L., Brown, C. M., and Gibson, P. J. (2004). Ethnicity and prescription patterns for haloperidol, risperidone, and olanzapine. *Psychiatric Services, 55(2)*, 151–56.

Orellana, R. T. (1989). Migratory movements and their effects on family structure: The Latin American case. *International Migration, 27(2)*, 319–32.

Ortega-Vélez, R. E. (1998). *Sobre violencia domestica* [About domestic violence]. San Juan, Puerto Rico: Ediciones Scisio.

Ortiz-Torres, B., Serrano-García, I., and Torres-Burgos, N. (2000). Subverting culture: Promoting HIV/AIDS prevention among Puerto Rican and Dominican women. *American Journal of Community Psychology, 28(6)*, 859–81.

O'Sullivan, M. J., and Lasso, B. (1992). Community mental health services for Hispanics: A test of the culture compatibility hypothesis. *Hispanic Journal of Behavioral Sciences, 14(4)*, 455–68.

Otto-Salaj, L. L., Heckman, J. G., Stevenson, L. Y., and Kelly, J. A. (1998). Patterns, predictors and gender differences in HIV risk among severely mentally ill men and women. *Community Mental Health Journal, 34(2)*, 175–90.

Oyserman, D., Mowbray, C. T., Meares, P. A., and Firminger, K. B. (2000). Parenting among mothers with a serious mental illness. *American Journal of Orthopsychiatry, 70(3)*, 296–315.

Padgett, D., Struening, E. L., and Andrews, H. (1990). Factors affecting the use of medical, mental health, alcohol, and drug treatment services by homeless adults. *Medical Care, 28*, 805–21.

Padian, N. S., Shiboski, S. C., Glass, S. O., and Vittinghoff, E. (1997). Heterosexual transmission of human immunodeficiency virus (HIV) in northern California: Results from a ten-year study. *American Journal of Epidemiology, 146(4)*, 350–57.

Padilla, F. M. (1990). Salsa: Puerto Rican and Latino music. *Journal of Popular Culture, 24*, 87–104.

Padilla, F. M. (1989). Salsa music as a cultural expression of Latino consciousness and unity. *Hispanic Journal of Behavioral Sciences, 11*, 28–45.

Panitz, D., McConchie, A., Sauber, S., and Fonseca, J. (1983). The role of machismo and the Hispanic family in the etiology and treatment of alcoholism in Hispanic

American men. *American Journal of Family Therapy, 11*, 31–44.
Parillo, K. M., Freeman, R. C., Collier, K., and Young, P. (2001). Association between early sexual abuse and adult HIV-risky sexual behaviors among community-based women. *Child Abuse and Neglect, 25*, 335–46.
Patron, M. G. (1969). La psicología del mexicano [The psychology of the Mexican male]. *Revista Mexicana de Psicología, 3*, 350–54.
Peñalosa, F. (1968). Mexican family roles. *Journal of Marriage and the Family, 30*, 680–89.
Perese, E. F. (2003). Stigma, poverty, and victimization: Roadblocks to recovery for individuals with severe mental illness. *Journal of the American Psychiatric Nurses Association, 13(5)*, 285–95.
Perese, E. F. (1997). Unmet needs of persons with chronic mental illnesses: Relationship to their adaptation to community living. *Issues in Mental Health Nursing, 18(1)*, 18–34.
Pérez-Jiménez, D., Cunningham, I., Serrano-García, I., and Ortiz-Torres, B. (2007). Construction of male sexuality and gender roles in Puerto Rican heterosexual college students. *Men and Masculinities, 9(3)*, 358–78.
Perez-Stable, E., Nápoles-Springer, A., and Miramontes, J. (1997). The effects of ethnicity and language on medical outcomes of patients with hypertension or diabetes. *Medical Care, 12*, 1212–19.
Perilla, J. L. (1999). Domestic violence as a human rights issue: The case of immigrant Latinos. *Hispanic Journal of Behavioral Sciences, 21*, 107–33.
Perilla, J. L., Bakeman, R., and Norris, F. H. (1994). Culture and domestic violence: The ecology of abused Latinas. *Violence and Victims, 9*, 325–39.
Perloff, H. (1950). *Puerto Rico's economic future*. Chicago: University of Chicago Press.
Phillips, R. E., III, Lakin, R., and Pargament, K. I. (2002). Development and implementation of a spiritual issues psychoeducational group for those with serious mental illness. *Community Mental Health Journal, 8(6)*, 487–95.
Pinto, R. M. (2005). Using social network interventions to improve mentally ill clients' well-being. *Clinical Social Work Journal, 34(1)*, 83–100.
Piore, M. (1979). *Birds of passage: Migrant labor and industrial societies*. New York: Cambridge University Press.
Platt, J. J. (1995). Vocational rehabilitation of drug abusers. *Psychology Bulletin, 117*, 416–33.
Plewes, J. M., II, Bailey, R. K., Mallinckrodt, C. H., Watkin, J. G., Wohlreich, M. M., and Lewis-Fernández, R. (2004). Duloxetine for the treatment of major depressive disorder in Hispanic and African American patients. Paper presented at the American Psychiatric Association Annual Meeting, New York, May 1–6.
Polak, P., and Warner, R. (1996). The economic life of seriously mentally ill people in the community. *Psychiatric Services, 47(2)*, 270–74.
Pribor, E. F., and Dinwiddie, S. H. (1992). Psychiatric correlates of incest in childhood. *American Journal of Psychiatry, 149*, 52–56.
Prochaska, J., and DiClemente, C. (1992). Stages of change in the modification of problem behaviors. In M. Hersen, R. Meisler, and P. M. Miller (Eds.). *Progress in behavior modification* (pp. 184–214). New York: Sycamore.
Prochaska, J., and DiClemente, C. (1984). *The transtheoretical approach: Crossing traditional boundaries of change*. Homewood, IL: Dorsey Press.
Purdon, S. E., Jones, B. D. W., Stip, E., Labelle, A., Addington, D., David, S. R., et al. (2000). Neuropsychological change in early phase schizophrenia during 12 months of treatment with olanzapine, risperidone, or haloperidol. *Archives of General Psychiatry, 57*, 249–58.
Quinlivan, R., Hough, R. L., Crowell, A., Beach, C., Hofstetter, R., and

Kenworthy, K. (1995). Service utilization and costs of care for severely mentally ill clients in an intensive case management program. *Psychiatric Services, 46*, 365–71.

Quinn, A. M. (2006). *A dictionary of psychology*, 2nd ed. New York: Oxford University Press.

Rabow, J., and Watt, R. (1982). Alcohol availability, alcohol beverage sales, and alcohol-related problems. *Journal of Studies on Alcohol, 43*, 767–801.

Raiteri, K., Fora, R., Gioannini, P., Russo, R., Lucchini, A., Terzi, M. G., Giacobbi, D., and Sinicco, A. (1994). Seroprevalence, risk factors, and attitudes to HIV-1 in a representative sample of lesbians in Turin. *Genitourinary Medicine, 70*, 200–205.

Ramlow, B. E., White, A. L., Watson, D. D., and Leukefeld, C. G. (1997). The needs of women with substance use problems: An expanded vision for treatment. *Substance Use and Misuse, 32*, 1395–1404.

Read, J., Agar, K., Argyle, N., and Aderhold, V. (2003). Sexual and physical abuse during childhood and adulthood as predictors of hallucinations, delusions, and though disorder. *Psychology and Psychotherapy: Theory, Research, and Practice, 76*, 1–22.

Reed, R. J., and Grant, I. (1990). The long-term neurobehavioral components of substance abuse: Conceptual and methodological challenges for future research. In *Residual effects of abused drugs on behavior* (National Institute on Drug Abuse Research Monograph No. 101, pp. 10–56). Washington, DC: National Institute on Drug Abuse.

Reeves, K. (1986). Hispanic utilization of an ethnic mental health clinic. *Journal of Psychosocial Nursing and Mental Health Services, 24(2)*, 23–26.

Regier, D. A., Framer, M. E., Rae, D. S., Locke, B. Z., Keith, S. J., Judo, L. L., and Goodwin, F. K. (1990). Comorbidity of mental disorders with alcohol and other drug abuse: Results from the Epidemiologic Catchment Area (ECA) Study. *Journal of the American Medical Association, 264*, 2511–18.

Reidpath, D. D., and Chan, K. Y. (2005). A method for the quantitative analysis of the layering of HIV-related stigma. *AIDS Care, 17(4)*, 425–32.

Rhodes, T., Singer, M., Bourgois, P., Friedman, S. R., and Strathdee, S. A. (2005). The social structural production of HIV risk among injecting drug users. *Social Science and Medicine, 61*, 1026–44.

Richards, B. (1983). The uncertain state of Puerto Rico. *National Geographic, 163(4)*, 516–42.

Richardson, A. (1974). *British immigrants and Australia: A psycho-social inquiry.* Canberra: Australian National University Press.

Richardson, D. (2000). The social construction of community: HIV risk perception and prevention among lesbians and bisexual women. *Culture, Health and Sexuality, 1*, 33–49.

Ridgeway, P., and Rapp, C. (1998). *The active ingredients in achieving competitive employment for people with psychiatric disabilities: A research synthesis.* Lawrence, KS: Commission on Mental Health and Developmental Disabilities.

Rinaldi, M., and Perkins, R. (2007). Vocational rehabilitation for people with mental health problems. *Psychiatry, 6*, 373–76.

Riskind, J. H., and Wahl, O. (1992). Moving makes it worse: The role of rapid movement in fear of psychiatric patients. *Journal of Social and Clinical Psychology, 11*, 349–64.

Riszt, K. (1979). Incest: Theoretical and clinical views. *American Journal of Orthopsychiatry, 49(4)*, 680–91.

Ritsher, J. B., and Phelan, J. C. (2004). Internalized stigma predicts erosion of morale among psychiatric patients. *Psychiatry Research, 129*, 257–65.

Rivera, E. G. (2005). La Colonia de Lorain, Ohio. In C. T. Whalen and V. Vázquez-Hernández (Eds.). *The Puerto Rican diaspora: Historical perspectives* (pp.

151–73). Philadelphia: Temple University Press.

Robertson, J. A., and Plant, M. A. (1988). Alcohol, sex, and risks of HIV infection. *Drug and Alcohol Dependence, 22*, 75–78.

Rodgers, K. B. (1999). Parenting processes related to sexual risk-taking behaviors of adolescent males and females. *Journal of Marriage and Family, 61*, 99–109.

Rodriguez, C. E. (1994). A summary of Puerto Rican migration to the United States. In G. Lamberty and C. Garcia Coll (Eds.). *Puerto Rican women and children: Issues in health, growth, and development* (pp. 11–28). New York: Plenum Press.

Rogers, E. M., and Antola, L. (1985). Telenovelas: A Latin American success story. *Journal of Communication, 35(4)*, 24–35.

Rogers, E. S., Sciarappa, K., McDonald-Wilson, K., and Danley, L. (1995). A benefit-cost analysis of supported employment model for persons with psychiatric disabilities. *Evaluation Program Planning, 18(2)*, 105–15.

Rogler, L. H., Malgady, R. G., Constantino, G., and Blumenthal, R. (1987). What do culturally sensitive mental health services mean? The case of Hispanics. *American Psychologist, 42*, 565–70.

Rogosh, R. A., Mowbray, C. T., and Bogat, G. A. (1992). Determinants of parenting attitudes in mothers with severe psychopathology. *Developmental Psychopathology, 4*, 460–87.

Román, D. (1995). Teatro Viva! Latino performance and the politics of AIDS in Los Angeles. In E. L. Bergmann and P. J. Smith (Eds.). *Entiendes? Queer Readings, Hispanic Writings* (pp. 346–69). Durham, NC: Duke University Press.

Romero-Daza, N., Weeks, M., and Singer, M. (2003). "Nobody gives a damn if I live or die": Violence, drugs, and street-level prostitution in inner-city Hartford, Connecticut. *Medical Anthropology, 22*, 233–59.

Rose, P. (1993). Out in the open? *Nursing Times, 89*, 50–52.

Rosen, M. I., McMahon, T. J., Lin, H. Q., and Rosenheck, R. A. (2006). Effect of Social Security payments on substance abuse in a homeless mentally ill cohort. *Health Services Research, 41*, 173–91.

Rosenberg, S. D., Lu, W., Mueser, K. T., Jankowski, M. K., and Cournos, F. (2007). Correlates of adverse childhood events among adults with schizophrenia spectrum disorders. *Psychiatric Services, 58*, 245–53.

Rosenfield, S. (1989). The effects of women's employment: Personal control and sex differences in mental health. *Journal of Health and Social Behavior, 30*, 77–91.

Rosenstock, I. M. (1974). Historical origins of the health belief model. In M. H. Becker (Ed.). *The health belief model and personal health behavior.* Thorofare, NY: Slack.

Ross, C. E., and Broh, B. A. (2000). The roles of self-esteem and the sense of personal control in the academic achievement process. *Sociology of Education, 73*, 270–84.

Rothaus, P., Hanson, P. G., Cleveland, S. E., and Johnson, D. L. (1964). Mental illness and employment [letter]. *American Psychologist, 19*, 200–201.

Rozensky, R. H., and Gomez, M. Y. (1983). Language switching in psychotherapy with bilinguals: Two problems, two models and case examples. *Psychotherapy: Theory, Research and Practice, 20*, 152–60.

Ruiz-Marrero, C. (2002). Puerto Ricans outraged over secret medical experiments. *Puerto Rico Herald*, Oct. 21. Retrieved March 25, 2009, from *puertorico-herald.org/issues/2002/vol6n44/PROutragMedExp-en.html.*

Rüsch, N., Angermeyer, M. C., and Corrigan, P. W. (2005). Mental illness stigma: Concepts, consequences, and initiatives to reduce stigma. *European Psychiatry, 20*, 529–39.

Rutter, M. (1990). The developmental psychopathology of depression: Issues and perspectives. In J. Rolf, A. S. Masten, D. Cicchetti, K. N. Nuechterlein, and S. Weintraub (Eds.). *Risk and protective factors in the development of psychopathology.* Cambridge: Cambridge University Press.

Ryan, W. (1976). *Blaming the victim*, rev. ed. New York: Random House.

Sabogal, F., Marín, G., Otero-Sabogal, R., Marín, B. V., and Perez-Stable, E. J. (1987). Hispanic familism and acculturation: What changes and what doesn't. *Hispanic Journal of Behavioral Sciences, 9(4)*, 397–412.

Sacks, M. H., and Dermatis, H. (1994). Acute psychiatric illness: Effects on HIV-risk behavior. *Psychosocial Rehabilitation Journal, 17*, 5–19.

Sacks, M. H., Dermatis, H., Looser-Ott, S., and Perry, S. (1992). Seroprevalence of HIV and risk factors for AIDS in psychiatric inpatients. *Hospital and Community Psychiatry, 43*, 736–37.

Sajatovic, M., and Ramirez, L. F. (2001). *Rating scales in mental health*. Hudson, OH: Lexi-Comp.

Salgado de Snyder, N., and Padilla, A. M. (1987). Social support networks: Their availability and effectiveness. In M. Gaviria and J. Arana (Eds.). *Health and behavior: Research agenda for Hispanics* (pp. 93–107). Simón Bolívar Research Monograph Series No. 1. Chicago: University of Illinois at Chicago.

Salmán, E., Liebowitz, M. R., Guarnaccia, P. J., Jusino, C. M., Garfinkel, R., Street, L., Cárdenas, D. L., Silvestre, J., Fyer, A. J., Carrasco, J. L., Davies, S. O., and Klein, D. F. (1998). Subtypes of ataques de nervios: The influence of co-existing psychiatric diagnoses. *Culture, Medicine, and Psychiatry, 22*, 231–44.

Sameroff, A., Seifer, R., and Zax, M. (1982). Early development of children at risk for emotional disorder. *Monographs in Social Research in Child Development, 47*(7, Serial No. 199).

Sánchez Korrol, V. (1983). *From colonia to community: The history of Puerto Ricans in New York City, 1917–1948*. Westport, CT: Greenwood Press.

Sánchez-Lacay, J. A., Lewis-Fernández, R., Goetz, D., Blanco, C., Salmán, E., Davies, S., et al. (2001). Open trial of nefazodone among Hispanics with major depression: Efficacy, tolerability, and adherence issues. *Depression and Anxiety, 13*, 118–24.

Santana, M. C., Raj, A., Decaer, M. R., La Marche, A., and Silverman, J. G. (2006). Masculine gender roles associated with increased sexual risk and intimate partner violence perpetration among young adult men. *Journal of Urban Health, 83(4)*, 575–85.

Santana Cooney, R., and Colon, A. (1996). Work and family: The recent struggle of Puerto Rican females. In C. E. Rodriguez and V. Sánchez Korrol (Eds.). *Historical perspectives on Puerto Rican survival in the United States* (pp. 70–85). Princeton, NJ: Markus Weiner.

Sartorius, N. (2007). Stigma and mental health. *Lancet, 370*, 810–11.

Schaef, A. W. (1987). *When society becomes an addict.* San Francisco: Harper and Row.

Scheff, T. J. (1984). *Being mentally ill: A sociological theory*, 2nd ed. New York: Aldine de Gruyler.

Scheff, T. J. (1966). *Being mentally ill: A sociological theory*. Chicago: Aldine.

Schoen, J. (2005). *Choice and coercion: Birth control, sterilization, and abortion in public health and welfare*. Chapel Hill: University of North Carolina Press.

Schulze, B., and Angermeyer, M. C. (2003). Subjective experiences of stigma: A focus group study of schizophrenic patients, their relatives and mental health professionals. *Social Science and Medicine, 56*, 299–312.

Schur, E. (1971). *Labeling deviant behavior*. New York: Harper and Row.

Schwalbe, M. L., and Staples, C. L. (1991). Gender differences in sources of self-esteem. *Psychology Quarterly, 54*, 158–68.

Schwartz-Watts, D., Montgomery, L. D., and Morgan, D. W. (1995). Seroprevalence of human immunodeficiency virus among inpatient pretrial detainees. *Bulletin of the American Academy of Psychiatry and Law, 23*, 285–88.

Seeman, M. V., and Cohen, R. (1998). Focus

on women: A service for women with schizophrenia. *Psychiatric Services, 49*, 674–77.

Sells, D. J., Rowe, M., Fisk, D., and Davidson, L. (2003). Violent victimization of persons with co-occurring psychiatric and substance use disorders. *Psychiatric Services, 54(9)*, 1253–57.

Senior, C., and Watkins, D. O. (1966). Toward a balance sheet of Puerto Rican migration. In *Status of Puerto Rico: Selected background studies for the United States-Puerto Rico Commission on the Status of Puerto Rico* (pp. 715–16). Washington, DC: U.S. Government Printing Office.

Senn, T. E., and Carey, M. P. (2008). HIV testing among individuals with a severe mental illness: Review, suggestions for research, and clinical implications. *Psychological Medicine, 39*, 355–63.

Silberstein, C., Galanter, M., Marmor, M., Lisshutz, H., and Krasinski, K. (1994). HIV-1 among inner city dually diagnosed inpatients. *American Journal of Drug and Alcohol Abuse, 20*, 101–31.

Simmons, J., and Singer, M. (2006). I love you . . . and heroin: Care and collusion among drug-using couple. *Substance Abuse Treatment, Prevention, and Policy, 1(1)*, 7. doi:10.1186/1747-597X-1-7.

Simon, W., and Gagnon, J. H. (1987). A sexual scripts approach. In J. H. Geer and W. O'Donahue (Eds.). *Theories of human sexuality* (pp. 363–83). New York: Plenum.

Simpson, T. L., and Miller, W. R. (2002). Concomitance between childhood sexual and physical abuse and substance use problems: A review. *Clinical Psychology Review, 22*, 27–77.

Sirey, J. A., Meters, B. S., Bruce, M. L., Alexopoulos, G. S., Perlick, D. A., and Raue, P. (1999). Predictors of antidepressant prescription and early use among depressed outpatients. *American Journal of Psychiatry, 156*, 690–96.

Sobell, M. B., Brochu, S., Sobell, L. C., Roy, J., and Stevens, J. A. (1987). Alcohol treatment outcome evaluation methodology: State of the art, 1980–1984. *Addictive Behaviors, 12*, 113–28.

Soto, E., and Shaver, P. (1982). Sex-role traditionalism, assertiveness, and symptoms of Puerto Rican women living in the United States. *Hispanic Journal of Behavioral Sciences, 4(1)*, 1–19.

Springer, K. W., Sheridan, J., Kuo, D., and Carnes, M. (2007). Long-term physical and mental health consequences of childhood physical abuse: Results from a large population-based sample of men and women. *Child Abuse and Neglect, 31*, 517–30.

Springs, F. E., and Friedrich, W. N. (1992). Health risk behaviors and medical sequelae of childhood sexual abuse. *Mayo Clinic Proceedings, 67*, 527–32.

Stall, R., McKusick, L., and Wiley, J. (1986). Alcohol and drug use during sexual activity: Compliance with safe sex for AIDS. *Health Education Quarterly, 13*, 359–71.

Stangor, C., and Ruble, D. N. (1989). Strength of expectancies and memory for social information: What we remember depends on how much we know. *Journal of Experimental Social Psychology, 25*, 18–35.

Star, S. (1955). The public's ideas about mental illness. Presented at the Annual Meeting of the National Association for Mental Health, November 5. Cited in Link, B. G., Phelan, J. C., Bresnahan, M., Stueve, A., and Pescosolido, B. A. (1999). Public conceptions of mental illness: Labels, causes, dangerousness, and social distance. *American Journal of Public Health, 89(9)*, 1328–33.

Steele, F. R. (1994). A moving target: CDC still trying to estimate HIV-1 prevalence. *Journal of NIH Research, 6*, 25–26.

Stein, J. A., Leslie, M. B., and Nyamathi, A. (2002). Relative contributions of parent substance use and childhood maltreatment to chronic homelessness, depression, and substance abuse problems among homeless women: Mediating roles of self-esteem and abuse in adulthood. *Child Abuse and Neglect, 26*, 1011–27.

Steiner, J., Lussier, R., and Rosenblatt, W. (1992). Knowledge about and risk factors for AIDS in a day hospital population. *Hospital and Community Psychiatry, 43*, 734–35.

Stevens, P. E. (1994). Lesbians and HIV: Clinical, research, and policy issues. *Journal of Orthopsychiatry, 63*, 289–95.

Stevens-Arroyo, A. M. (2000). Catholicism's emerging role in Puerto Rico. *America, 182(13)*, 8–11.

Stevens-Arroyo, A. M., and Diaz-Stevens, M. (1982). Puerto Ricans in the United States: A struggle for identity. In A. G. Dworkin and R. J. Dworkin (Eds.). *The minority report: Introduction to racial, ethnic, and gender relations*. New York: Holt, Rinehart and Winston.

Stewart, D. L., Zuckerman, C. J., and Ingle, J. M. (1994). HIV seroprevalence in a chronically mentally ill population. *Journal of the National Medical Association, 86*, 519–23.

Stott, F. M., Musick, J. S., Cohler, B. J., Spencer, K. K., Goldman, J., Clark, R., and Dincin, J. (1984). Intervention for the severely disturbed mother. In J. Musick and B. Cohler (Eds.). *Intervention among psychiatrically impaired parents and their young children* (pp. 7–32). San Francisco: Jossey-Bass.

Straus, M. A. (2001). *Beating the devil out of them: Corporal punishment in American families and its effects on children.* New Brunswick, NJ: Transaction.

Straus, M. A. (1991). Discipline and deviance: Physical punishment of children and violence and other crimes in adulthood. *Social Problems, 38*, 101–23.

Straus, M. A., and Kantor, G. (1994). Corporal punishment of adolescents by parents: A risk factor in the epidemiology of depression, suicide, alcohol abuse, child abuse, and wife beating. *Adolescence, 29(115)*, 543–62.

Sue, S., Fujino, D. C., Hu, L., and Takeuchi, D. T. (1991). Community mental health services for ethnic minority groups: A test of the cultural responsiveness hypothesis. *Journal of Consulting and Clinical Psychology, 59*, 533–40.

Sullivan, W. P. (1998). Recoiling, regrouping, and recovering: First-person accounts of the role of spirituality in the course of serious mental illness. *New Directions for Mental Health Services, 80*, 25–33.

Susser, E., Valencia, E., and Conover, S. (1993). Prevalence of HIV infection among psychiatric patients in a New York City men's shelter. *American Journal of Public Health, 83*, 568–70.

Suyemoto, K. L., and MacDonald, M. L. (1995). Self-cutting in female adolescents. *Psychotherapy, 32(1)*, 162–71.

Swanson, J. W., Swartz, M. S., Essock, S. M., Osher, F. C., Wagner, R., Goodman, L. A., Rosenberg, S. D., and Meador, K. G. (2002). The social-environmental context of violent behavior in persons treated for severe mental illness. *American Journal of Public Health, 92(9)*, 1523–31.

Swartz, M. S., Swanson, J. W., Hiday, V. A., Borum, R., Wagner, R., and Burns, B. J. (1998). Violence and severe mental illness: The effects of substance abuse a nd nonadherence to medication. *American Journal of Psychiatry, 155(2)*, 226–31.

Talwar, N., Crawford, M. J., Maratos, A., Nur, U., McDermott, O., and Procter, S. (2006). Music therapy for in-patients with schizophrenia: Exploratory randomized controlled trial. *British Journal of Psychiatry, 189*, 405–9.

Tang, W., Yao, X., and Zheng, Z. (1994). Rehabilitative effect of music therapy for residual schizophrenia: A one-month randomized controlled trial in Shanghai. *British Journal of Psychiatry, Suppl. 24*, 38–44.

Tanskanen, A., Hintikka, J., Honkalampi, K., Haatainenk, K., Koivumaa-Honkanen, H., and Viinamäki, H. (2004). Impact of multiple traumatic experiences on the persistence of depressive symptoms—A population-based study. *Nordic Journal of Psychiatry, 58(6)*, 459–64.

Tashakkori, A., and Teddlie, C. (1998). *Mixed methodology: Combining qualitative and quantitative approaches.* Applied Social Research Methods Series, vol. 46. Thousand Oaks, CA: Sage.

Taylor, S. M., and Dear, M. J. (1981). Scaling community attitudes toward the mentally ill. *Schizophrenia Bulletin, 7*, 225–40.

Tepper, L., Rogers, S. A., Coleman, E. M., and Malony, H. N. (2001). The prevalence of religious coping among persons with persistent mental illness. *Psychiatric Services, 52(5)*, 660–65.

Test, M. A. (1998). Community-based treatment models for adults with severe and persistent mental illness. In J. B. W. Williams and K. Ell (Eds.). *Recent advances in mental health research: Implications for practice* (pp. 420–36). Washington, DC: NASW Press.

Thaut, M. H. (1990). Neuropsychological processes in music perception and their relevance in music therapy. In R. F. Unkefer (Ed.). *Music therapy in the treatment of adults with mental disorders* (pp. 3–32). New York: Schirmer.

Thomson, W., Jr. (2005). *Getting in the door: Language barriers to health services at New York City's hospitals.* New York: New York City Comptroller, Office of Policy Management.

Tolsdorf, C. C. (1976). Social networks, support, and coping: An exploratory study. *Family Process, 15*, 407–18.

Torres, A., and Velazquez, J. E. (1998). *The Puerto Rican movement: Voices from the diaspora.* Philadelphia: Temple University Press.

Torres, S. (1991). A comparison of wife abuse between two cultures: Perceptions, attitudes, nature, and extent. *Issues in Mental Health Nursing, 12*, 113–31.

Torres-Matrullo, C. (1982). Cognitive therapy of depressive disorders in the Puerto Rican female. In R. M. Becerra, M. Karno, and J. I. Escobar (Eds.). *Mental health and Hispanic Americans* (pp. 101–13). New York: Grune & Stratton.

Torrey, F. E., and Knable, M. B. (2002). *Surviving manic depression: A manual on bipolar disorder for patients, families and providers.* New York: Guilford Press.

Triandis, H. C., Marín, G., Betancourt, H., Lisansky, J., and Chang, B. (1982). Dimensions of familism among Hispanic and mainstream Navy recruits, 1982. Cited in Marín, G. (1993). Influence of acculturation on familism and self-identification among Hispanics. In G. Knight and M. Bernal (Eds.). *Ethnic identity: Formation and transmission among Hispanics and other minorities.* New York: State University of New York Press.

Twitchell, G. R., Hertzong, C. A., Klein, J. L., and Schuckit, M. A. (1992). The anatomy of a follow-up. *British Journal of Addiction, 87*, 1327–33.

U.S. Census Bureau. (2008a). American factfinder: Fact sheet: Cuyahoga County, Ohio. Retrieved September 13, 2010, from *factfinder.census.gov/servlet/SAFFacts?_event=ChangeGeoContext&_county=Cuyahoga&_state=040004539.*

U.S. Census Bureau. (2008b). State and county quickfacts: Cuyahoga County, Ohio. Retrieved August 13, 2008, from *quickfacts.census.gov/qfd/states/39/39035.html.*

U.S. Census Bureau. (2005). U.S. Census Bureau news. Retrieved April 6, 2009, from *www.census.gov/Press-Release/www/releases/archives/income_wealth/005647.html.*

U.S. Commission on Civil Rights. (1976). *Puerto Ricans in the continental United States: An uncertain future.* Washington, DC: U.S. Commission on Civil Rights.

U.S. Department of Agriculture. (2006). Nutrition program facts: Food and nutrition service: WIC. Retrieved April 6, 2009, from *www.fns.uda.gov/WIC-Fact-Sheet.pdf.*

U.S. Department of Health and Human Services. (2001). *Mental health: Culture, race, and ethnicity: A supplement to mental health: A report of the surgeon general.* Rockville, MD: U.S. Department of Health and Human Services.

U.S. Department of Housing and Urban Development. (2005). *The state of the cities—1998: Part one: The state of America's cities.* Washington, DC: U.S. Department of Housing and Urban Development. Retrieved September 13, 2010, from *www.huduser.org/Publications/PDF/soc_98.pdf.*

U.S. Department of Housing and Urban Development. (2004). Section 8 rental voucher program. Retrieved April 6, 2009, from *www.hud.gov/progdesc/voucher.cfm.*

U.S. Drug Enforcement Administration. (2010). Oxycontin. Retrieved September 13, 2010, from *www.justice.gov/dea/concern/oxycontin.html.*

U.S. Government Accountability Office. (2009). *Report to congressional committees: Ryan White Care Act: Implementation of the new Minority AIDS Provisions.* GAO-09-315. Washington, DC: U.S. Government Accountability Office.

Valenzuela, S. M., and Dornbusch, S. M. (1994). Familism and social capital in the academic achievement of Mexican origin and Anglo adolescents. *Social Science Quarterly, 75*, 18–36.

Valois, R. F., Bryant, E. S., Rivard, J. C., and Hinkle, K. T. (1997). Sexual risk-taking behavior among adolescents with severe emotional disturbance. *Journal of Child and Family Studies, 6*, 409–19.

Van Dorn, R. A., Mustillo, S., Elbogen, E. B., Dorsey, S., Swanson, J. W., and Swartz, M. S. (2005). The effects of early sexual abuse on adult risky sexual behaviors among persons with severe mental illness. *Child Abuse and Neglect, 29*, 1265–79.

Vandello, J. A., and Cohen, D. (2003). Male honor and female fidelity: Implicit cultural scripts that perpetuate domestic violence. *Journal of Personality and Social Psychology, 84(5)*, 997–1010.

Vasquez, M. J. T. (1998). Latinas and violence: Mental health implications and strategies for clinicians. *Cultural Diversity and Mental Health, 4*, 319–34.

Vega, W. A., and Alegría, M. (2001). Latino mental health and treatment in the United States. In M. Aguirre-Molina, C. Molina, and R. Zambrana (Eds.). *Health issues in the Latino community* (pp. 179–208). San Francisco: Jossey-Bass.

Vega, W. A., and Lopez, S. R. (2001). Priority issues in Latino mental health services research. *Mental Health Services Research, 3(4)*, 189–200.

Ventura, S. J. (1994). Demographic and health characteristics of Puerto Rican mothers and their babies, 1990. In G. Lamberty and C. Garcia Coll (Eds.). *Puerto Rican women and children: Issues in health, growth, and development* (pp. 71–84). New York: Plenum.

Verdejo-García, A. J., López-Torrecillas, F., Aguilar de Arcos, F., and Pérez-García, M. (2005). Differential effects of MDMA, cocaine, and cannabis use severity on distinctive components of the executive functions in polysubstance users: A multiple regression analysis. *Addictive Behaviors, 30(1)*, 89–101.

Villarruel, A. M., Jemmott, J. B., and Jemmott, L. S. (2006). A randomized controlled trial testing an HIV prevention intervention for Latino youth. *Archives of Pediatrics and Adolescent Medicine, 160*, 772–77.

Volavka, J., Convit, A., Czobor, P., Dwyer, R., O'Donnell, J., Jr., and Ventura, A. (1991). HIV seroprevalence and risk behaviors in psychiatric inpatients. *Psychiatry Research, 39*, 109–14.

Wagenheim, K., and Jiménez de Wagenheim, O. (Eds.). (1994). *The Puerto Ricans: A documentary history.* Princeton, NJ: Marcus Wiener.

Wahl, O. F. (1999). Mental health consumers' experience of stigma. *Schizophrenia Bulletin, 25(3)*, 467–78.

Wahl, O. F. (1995). *Media madness: Public images of mental illness.* New Brunswick, NJ: Rutgers University Press.

Wahl, O. F., Wood, A., and Richards, R.

(2002). Newspaper coverage of mental illness: Is it changing? *Psychiatric Rehabilitation Skills, 6(1)*, 9–31.

Walker, L. E. (1978). Battered women and learned helplessness. *Victimology, 2*, 525–34.

Wang, P. S., Berglund, P., and Kessler, R. C. (2000). Recent care of common disorders in the United States: Prevalence and conformance with evidence-based recommendations. *Journal of General Internal Medicine, 15*, 284–92.

Ward, J. (2004). "Not all differences are created equal": Multiple jeopardy in a gendered organization. *Gender and Society, 18*, 82–102.

Warner, R., and Polak, P. (1995). The economic advancement of the mentally ill in the community: 2. Economic choices and disincentives. *Community Mental Health Journal, 31*, 477–92.

Waxman, M. A., and Levitt, M. A. (2000). Are diagnostic testing and admission rates higher in non-English-speaking versus English-speaking patients in the emergency department? *Annals of Emergency Medicine, 36*, 456–61.

Wegsheider-Cruse, S. (1985). *Choice-making*. Deerfield Beach, FL: Health Communications.

Weinberger, D. R. (1987). Implications of normal brain development for pathogenesis of schizophrenia. *Archives of General Psychiatry, 44*, 660–69.

Weinhardt, L. S., Carey, M. P., and Carey, K. B. (1998). HIV-risk behavior and the public health context of HIV/AIDS among women living with a severe and persistent mental illness. *Journal of Nervous and Mental Disease, 186*, 276–82.

Weinhardt, L. S., Carey, M. P., Carey, K. B., Maisto, S. C., and Gordon, C. M. (2001). The relation of alcohol use to HIV-risk sexual behavior among adults with severe and persistent mental illness. *Journal of Consulting and Clinical Psychology, 69*, 77–84.

Weinhardt, L. S., Carey, M. P., Carey, K. B., and Verdecias, R. N. (1998). Increasing assertiveness skills to reduce HIV risk among women living with a severe and persistent mental illness. *Journal of Consulting and Clinical Psychology, 66(4)*, 680–84.

Weisman, A. G. (2005). Integrating culturally based approaches with existing interventions for Hispanic/Latino families coping with schizophrenia. *Psychotherapy: Theory, Research, Practice, Training, 42(2)*, 178–97.

Weisman, A. G., Rosales, G., Kymalainen, J., and Armesto, J. (2005). Ethnicity, family cohesion, religiosity, and general emotional distress in patients with schizophrenia and their relatives. *Journal of Nervous and Mental Disease, 193(6)*, 359–68.

Weisman de Mamani, A. G., Rosales, G. Kymalainen, J., and Armesto, J. (2007). Expressed emotion and interdependence in white and Latino/Hispanic family members of patients with schizophrenia. *Psychiatry Research, 151*, 107–13.

Weisner, C., and Schmidt, L. (1992). Gender disparities in treatment for alcohol problems. *Journal of the American Medical Association, 268*, 1872–76.

Wells, K., Guo, S., Shafran, R., and Pearlmutter, S. (2003). Deterioration of child welfare families under conditions of welfare reform. Working paper. Chicago: University of Chicago. Retrieved April 29, 2009, from *www.jcpr.org/wpfiles/wells.pdf*.

Wells, K., Miranda, J., Bruce, M. L., Alegria, M., and Wallerstein, N. (2004). Bridging community intervention and mental health services research. *American Journal of Psychiatry, 161(6)*, 955–63.

Wenninger, K., and Ehlers, A. (1998). Dysfunctional cognitions and adult psychological functioning in child sexual abuse survivors. *Journal of Traumatic Stress, 11*, 231–300.

West, C. M. (1998). Lifting the "political gag order": Breaking the silence around partner violence in ethnic minority families. In J. L. Jasinski and L. M. Williams (Eds.). *Partner violence: A comprehensive review of 20 years of research* (pp. 184–209). Thousand Oaks, CA: Sage.

Whalen, C. T. (2005). Colonialism, citizenship, and the Puerto Rican diaspora. In C. T. Whalen and V. Vázquez-Hernández (Eds.). *The Puerto Rican diaspora: Historical perspectives* (pp. 1–42). Philadelphia: Temple University Press.

Williams, D. R., and Collins, C. (2001). Racial residential segregation: A fundamental cause of racial disparities in health. *Public Health Reports, 116*, 404–16.

Wilson, W. J. (1987). *The truly disadvantaged: The inner city, the underclass, and public policy*. Chicago: University of Chicago Press.

Wolfe, D. A. (1999). *Child abuse: Implications for child development and psychopathology*, 2nd ed. Thousand Oaks, CA: Sage.

Wong, Y. L. I., and Solomon, P. L. (2002). Community integration of persons with psychiatric disabilities in supportive independent housing: A conceptual model and methodological considerations. *Mental Health Services Research, 4(1)*, 13–28.

World Health Organization. (2001). *Mental health problems: The undefined and hidden burden*. Fact Sheet No. 218. Retrieved August 8, 2007, from *www.who.int/mediacentre/factsheets/fs218/eng/print.html.*

Wright, E. R., Gronfein, W. P., and Owens, T. J. (2000). Deinstitutionalization, social rejection, and the self-esteem for former mental patients. *Journal of Health and Social Behavior, 41*, 68–90.

Young, A. S., Chinman, M. J., Cradock-O'Leary, J. A., Sullivan, G., Murata, D., Mintz, J., and Koegel, P. (2005). Characteristics of individuals with severe mental illness who use emergency services. *Community Mental Health Journal, 41(2)*, 159–68.

Young, A. S., Klap, R., Sherbourne, C. D., and Wells, K. B. (2001). The quality of care for depressive and anxiety disorders in the United States. *Archives of General Psychiatry, 58*, 55–61.

Zea, M. C., Mason, M. A., and Murguia, A. (2000). Psychotherapy with members of Latino/Latina religions and spiritual traditions. In P. S. Richards and B. E. Allen (Eds.). *Handbook of psychotherapy and religious diversity* (pp. 397–419). Washington, DC: American Psychological Association.

Index

The letter *t* or *f* following a page number denotes a table or figure.

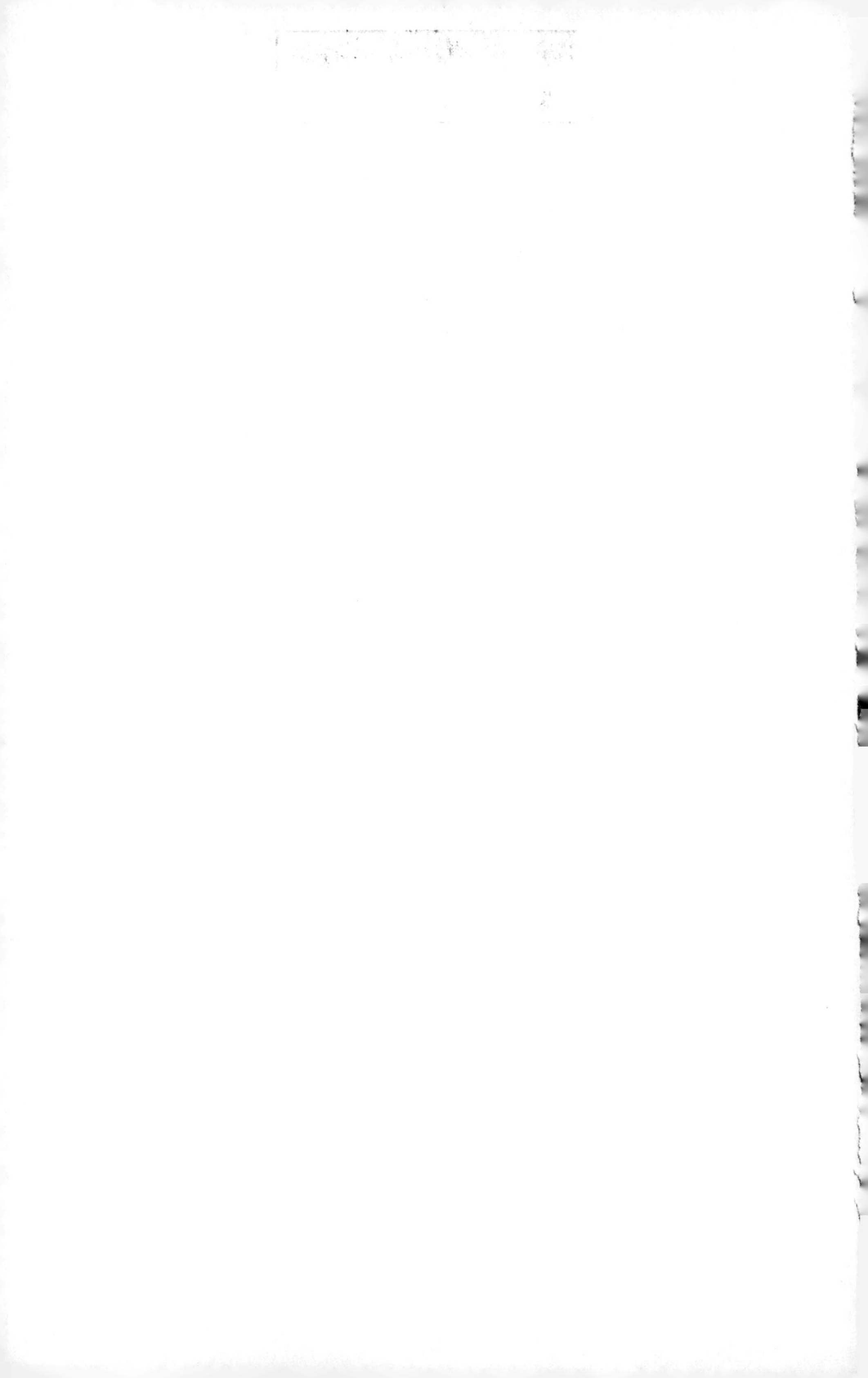